AMERICAN SIGN LANGUAGE FOR BEGINNERS

YOUR COMPREHENSIVE GUIDE TO RAPIDLY LEARNING ASL, FROM BASICS TO ADVANCED CONVERSATIONS - EFFECTIVE TECHNIQUES FOR FAST LEARNING

THE ASL ACADEMY

Copyright 2023 by The ASL Academy – All right reserved

This publication is protected by copyright. No part of this publication may be distributed or reproduced, including photocopying or other methods, without a signed permission of the owner. However, brief quotations, including critical reviews and other noncommercial uses permitted by copyright law, may be used with proper citation.

The contents of this book are intended solely for general information purposes. Although we do our best to ensure that the information in this book is accurate and current, we cannot guarantee its completeness, reliability, or suitability for any purpose. The information in the book is provided without any warranties. Any decision you make based on this information is at your own risk.

We shall not be held responsible for any loss or damage, including but not limited to indirect or consequential loss or damage, arising from the use of this book.

We strive to ensure the book runs smoothly, but we are not responsible for any temporary unavailability of the book due to factors outside our control. We hope you find the book enjoyable and appreciate your respect for the author's hard work.

TABLE OF CONTENTS

BOOK 1: FUNDAMENTALS OF ASL...5
    CHAPTER 1: INTRODUCTION TO AMERICAN SIGN LANGUAGE (ASL)...5
    CHAPTER 2: HISTORY AND EVOLUTION OF ASL..................6
    CHAPTER 3: MYTHS AND MISCONCEPTIONS ABOUT ASL...7
    CHAPTER 4: UNDERSTANDING THE BASICS: GESTURES, EXPRESSIONS, AND MOVEMENTS 8
    CHAPTER 5: THE ROLE OF FACIAL EXPRESSIONS AND BODY LANGUAGE...9
    CHAPTER 6: HOW TO STRUCTURE A SENTENCE 11
    CHAPTER 7: MASTERY OF THE ASL ALPHABET: A VISUAL GUIDE.. 14
    CHAPTER 8: LEARNING NUMBERS IN ASL 15
    CHAPTER 9: PRACTICAL EXERCISES: SPELLING WORDS AND NUMBERS 17
BOOK 2: BASIC CONVERSATIONS IN ASL............................. 18
    CHAPTER 1: ESSENTIAL SIGNS FOR DAILY COMMUNICATION 18
    CHAPTER 2: INTRODUCING YOURSELF AND MAKING CONVERSATION 27
    CHAPTER 3: GREETINGS, FAREWELLS, AND EVERYDAY PHRASES... 31
    CHAPTER 4: SIGNS FOR FAMILY MEMBERS AND RELATIONSHIPS 40
    CHAPTER 5: TIME AND DATES IN ASL................................... 45
    CHAPTER 6: BUILDING VOCABULARY: ADJECTIVES AND ADVERBS IN ASL 48
    CHAPTER 7: SIGNS FOR COMMON ACTIVITIES AND HOBBIES 51
    CHAPTER 8: FOOD AND BEVERAGES: FROM GROCERY SHOPPING TO DINING OUT.. 54
    CHAPTER 9: SEASONS, WEATHER, AND NATURE-RELATED SIGNS... 58
BOOK 3: ADVANCED SKILLS IN ASL... 61
    CHAPTER 1: DESCRIBING PEOPLE: APPEARANCE AND PERSONALITY 61
    CHAPTER 2: NAVIGATING: DIRECTIONS, PLACES, AND TRANSPORTATION 64
    CHAPTER 3: PLANNING EVENTS AND ACTIVITIES 66
    CHAPTER 4: AGREEING AND DISAGREEING IN ASL.......... 69

CHAPTER 5: EXPRESSING LIKES, DISLIKES, AND PREFERENCES 71
CHAPTER 6: INTERROGATIVE WORDS AND FORMULATING QUESTIONS IN ASL................................ 73
CHAPTER 7: UNDERSTANDING AND USING NON-MANUAL MARKERS FOR CLARITY.. 75

BOOK 4: PRACTICAL AND FUNCTIONAL ASL 77
CHAPTER 1: SIGNS FOR EMERGENCY SITUATIONS AND HEALTH... 77
CHAPTER 2: SIGN LANGUAGE IN EDUCATION AND THE WORKPLACE 80
CHAPTER 3: SIGNS FOR SHOPPING, MONEY, AND TRANSACTIONS 82
CHAPTER 4: PROVIDING INSTRUCTIONS AND DIRECTIONS 85
CHAPTER 5: PRACTICE STRATEGIES AND LEARNING RESOURCES 89
CHAPTER 6: INTERACTING WITH THE DEAF COMMUNITY 91
CHAPTER 7: OVERCOMING COMMON CHALLENGES AND FRUSTRATIONS 92

BOOK 5: INSIGHTS AND ADVANCED TOPICS IN ASL 94
CHAPTER 1: INTRODUCTION TO ASL GRAMMAR AND SYNTAX 94
CHAPTER 2: UNDERSTANDING IDIOMS AND PHRASES IN ASL... 95
CHAPTER 3: FREQUENTLY ASKED QUESTIONS ABOUT LEARNING ASL 97
CHAPTER 4: REFLECTIONS ON YOUR ASL JOURNEY 100
CHAPTER 5: BONUS: TIPS FOR FAST AND EFFECTIVE LEARNING 101
CHAPTER 6: CONCLUSIONS 104

BOOK 1: FUNDAMENTALS OF ASL
CHAPTER 1: INTRODUCTION TO AMERICAN SIGN LANGUAGE (ASL)

American Sign Language (ASL) is a dynamic language rich in expression, culture, and history that offers much more than just a means of communication. ASL conveys meaning through hand gestures, body language, and facial emotions as opposed to spoken languages. This makes it an exciting and visually stimulating method to communicate with others.

The power of ASL to eliminate barriers between the Deaf and hearing communities is at its core. It serves as many people's main source of communication and is necessary for daily interactions and information access. Others use it for interaction with relatives, close companions, or colleagues who are Deaf or hard of hearing. ASL is essentially a language that represents accessibility and unity.

Memorizing signs is only one aspect of learning ASL. It's about realizing a fresh perspective on the world and how to communicate ideas. The first step in exploring ASL is to recognize that it has a distinct structure that sets it apart from spoken languages. Meanings in American Sign Language (ASL) are expressed by body postures, facial emotions, and hand forms and gestures. The multifaceted nature of ASL communication renders it a demanding and captivating language to acquire.

You'll learn as you go along that ASL is a language unto itself; it is not influenced by English or any other spoken language. Its syntax, terms, and grammar are unique. This indicates that ASL is a language with its own characteristics and conventions rather than just a way to translate English into gestures. You will gain knowledge of the structure of ASL sentences, the meaning of signs, and how expressions and body language can change a phrase's meaning.

Learning the manual alphabet and numbers so that you can spell words and communicate numbers is one of the first steps in learning ASL. On top of these fundamental components, more intricate discussions can be constructed. As you advance, you'll pick up signs for commonplace tasks, descriptions, feelings, and more, allowing you to participate in a variety of conversations.

ASL's expressiveness and capacity to portray minute details of purpose and emotion are what make it so beautiful. You can communicate complicated ideas, jokes, and stories in ASL equally as well as, if not more successfully, than in spoken languages. You'll discover that ASL offers a rich, full-bodied form of expression because it is a language of the hands, face, and body as well.

Learning ASL provides an opportunity to fully immerse oneself in the history and culture of the Deaf community, in addition to its practical applications. You'll discover how ASL has been essential to the empowerment and campaigning for rights and recognition of Deaf people, as well as their struggles and victories.

As you immerse yourself in this book, keep in mind that learning ASL is a process that extends beyond picking up new abilities. It's an investigation into a multifaceted cultural fabric, a test of empathy, and a move in the direction of a more accepting society. This book will walk you through the fascinating world of American Sign Language, whether you're learning it to communicate with a Deaf family member, improve your professional skills, or just to explore a different culture.

CHAPTER 2: HISTORY AND EVOLUTION OF ASL

American Sign Language (ASL) is a rich texture that tells a meaningful and captivating story. This chapter on the "History and Evolution of ASL" explores the language's beginnings, following its path to important turning points that have molded it into the dynamic language it is today.

The official beginning of ASL was marked by the founding of the American School for the Deaf (ASD) in Hartford, Connecticut, in 1817. Deaf students from all over the country came together for this historic event, each bringing their own signs from home. These various signs came together to form the early basis of ASL, along with the impact of French Sign Language, which Thomas Hopkins Gallaudet learnt from Laurent Clerc. The foundation for the spread of ASL was created by Gallaudet's commitment and Clerc's instructional strategies, which eventually led to the establishment of several deaf schools around the nation, the majority of which were started by Clerc's students.

Thanks in large part to the influence of Thomas Hopkins Gallaudet's youngest son Edward Miner Gallaudet, there were notable advancements in deaf education throughout the mid-19th century. Following in his father's footsteps, Edward was instrumental in founding the National Deaf-Mute College in 1864, which went on to become Gallaudet College and, eventually, Gallaudet University. This university became a testing ground for ASL research and development in addition to offering the deaf community access to higher education.

William Stokoe, a professor of hearing at Gallaudet University and researcher, played a pivotal role in the history of ASL in 1960. Stokoe's dissertation demonstrated that ASL is a real language with its own syntax and grammar, which completely changed people's perceptions of it. By dispelling myths and paving the way for more linguistic research and advocacy, the acceptance of ASL as a valid language was a significant advancement.

Thanks to Laurent Clerc, the origins of ASL can be found in Old French Sign Language (LSF). But as time went on, ASL changed enough to set itself off from its French forebear by creating its own vocabulary, syntax, and grammar. This discrepancy illustrates how dynamic languages are, evolving and adapting to the unique cultural and social environments in which they are used.

The history of ASL is not merely linguistic; it is intricately linked to the social and cultural development of the American deaf population. ASL has developed from a means of basic communication to a symbol of pride and identity for the deaf population. It has been essential in promoting the rights of the deaf people, guaranteeing their educational opportunities, and helping them feel like they belong.

ASL's history is one of tenacity, inventiveness, and empowerment. ASL has played a crucial role in the deaf community's quest for self-expression and acceptance, from its beginnings at the American School for the Deaf to its acceptance as a full-fledged language. Knowing this past is more than just tracking a language's development; it's about appreciating and recognizing the diverse cultural fabric of the deaf community and the essential role that ASL plays in it.

CHAPTER 3: MYTHS AND MISCONCEPTIONS ABOUT ASL

There are many myths and misconceptions about American Sign Language. Not only do these false assumptions distort the fundamentals of ASL, but they also affect how the Deaf community is viewed and included in larger social conversations.

There is a widespread misperception that ASL is merely handwritten English that is meant to resemble spoken language. This is a basic misunderstanding. ASL is a unique language system that is very different from English or any other spoken language. It has its own syntax, grammar, and expressive nuances. Its composition is a distinct spatial and gestural assemblage of concepts rather than a translation of English words in a sequential fashion.

The notion that ASL is universal is another prevalent misconception. Sign languages are actually as varied as spoken languages, with variations found throughout various nations and areas. The rich cultural and linguistic legacy of the Deaf populations around the world is reflected in this differences.

The idea that ASL is an easier language to learn and a less complex option than spoken languages is a third common misunderstanding. This undervalues ASL's richness and complexity. Acquiring proficiency in ASL necessitates the same commitment and immersion as learning any other language, requiring knowledge of syntax, grammar, and cultural background.

There's also the notion that ASL has limited expressive power and can't explain complicated or abstract concepts. This misconception is untrue; ASL is a strong language that can convey a wide range of ideas, from tangible to abstract, and it's employed in a variety of contexts, such as academics and literature.

Finally, there is a misperception about the role that ASL plays in digital accessibility. Some people don't think ASL is necessary for digital inclusiveness. Nonetheless, the incorporation of sign language into digital systems is vital to guarantee complete accessibility. Ensuring effective communication and inclusivity while improving the internet experience for Deaf people is equally as important as adhering to accessibility guidelines.

These misconceptions not only distort perceptions of ASL, but they also make it more difficult to acknowledge the linguistic rights of the Deaf population. Clearing up these misunderstandings is essential to promoting an informed and inclusive view of ASL and Deaf culture.

CHAPTER 4: UNDERSTANDING THE BASICS: GESTURES, EXPRESSIONS, AND MOVEMENTS

Beyond basic hand movements, American Sign Language (ASL) is a visually expressive language. To communicate meaning, it uses a sophisticated system of both manual and non-manual components. It takes a thorough knowledge of these components and their subtle variations to comprehend the fundamentals.

- **Handshapes**: ASL employs distinct hand shapes, each of which stands for a particular letter, number, or idea. The way a sign is held can completely alter its meaning. For example, 'mother' and 'father' signify the same thing in the same place, but with distinct hand shapes.
- **Palm Orientation**: Determined by the direction the palm is facing when signing, the connotation can change. For instance, the arm motions used to indicate "enter" and "exit" are similar, but the palm faces different directions.
- **Movements**: ASL movements can depict objects, convey abstract

concepts, and indicate activities. They can be basic or complicated. A sharp movement, on the other hand, can represent urgency or suddenness. For example, a circular movement might describe something that happens again.
- **Facial Expressions**: Facial expressions in ASL are essential grammatical elements as well as emotive expressions. A furrowed brow is employed for WH-questions (who, what, where, when, and why), whereas raised eyebrows can transform a statement into a yes-or-no question.
- **Eye Gazing**: In ASL, eye contact is essential. It indicates engagement and denotes the start and finish of a turn in signing or a discussion.
- **Mouth Shapes**: Certain ASL signs require specific mouth shapes that correspond with the sign's meaning, which can be completely different from mouthing English words.
- **Body Posture and Movement**: The subject and object of a statement, as well as spatial links, can be shown by the signer's body alignment. While leaning back could represent past tense, leaning forward somewhat could indicate future tense.
- **Role Shifting**: This is moving one's head or body in order to represent several characters or points of view during a dialogue or story.
- **Use of Space**: ASL utilizes the area surrounding the signer. Signs placed in different points can symbolize various persons or things in space, forming a visual diagram of the communication.
- **Temporal Aspects**: Sign language's rhythm and pace might affect its meaning. A slow sign can suggest a prolonged length, whereas a fast sign might suggest a speedy action.

Communicating in ASL effectively requires an understanding of these components working together. It's a language that calls for body language and face expressiveness in addition to manual dexterity. Before going on to more complicated ideas, beginners should first become acquainted with basic hand shapes, gestures, and face expressions. The rich and complex linguistic system of ASL can be learned and understood much better via practice and immersion in the Deaf community.

CHAPTER 5: THE ROLE OF FACIAL EXPRESSIONS AND BODY LANGUAGE

Because American Sign Language (ASL) is a rich and intricate language that primarily uses visual clues, body language and facial expressions are essential for efficient communication. ASL uses body language and facial expressions to convey emphasis and emotions, in opposition to spoken languages where tone and volume play similar functions.

In ASL, facial expressions are essential grammatical elements of the language, not just emotional responses. Particular to sign languages, facial expressions play a grammatical function that is essential to understanding sentence meaning. Misunderstandings may result from misinterpreting or ignoring these facial cues since the meaning of a sign can vary depending on the facial expression that goes with it.

Beyond simple demonstrations of emotion, ASL facial gestures can convey subtleties in duration, intensity, and even rhetorical inquiries. The degree or seriousness of a thought being signed can be inferred from an intense or drawn-out expression. For instance, adding intensity to a basic "happy" facial expression might make it appear "ecstatic." Similar to this, rhetorical queries in ASL are frequently denoted by a particular facial expression, which typically consists of a head tilt that is slightly forward along with raised eyebrows.

In ASL, body language also conveys a lot of information. It can be used to express the movements and actions of persons or things, as well as to indicate where objects are located within the signing space. In ASL, since signs are frequently directional and their meaning can vary depending on which way they are signed, the utilization of space surrounding the signer is an essential component. A person or a thing, for example, can be represented by pointing to a space, and that person or object can then be further represented by using that space later in the discourse.

Additionally, body shifting in ASL is employed to portray many characters in a story. A small body turn combined with a change in expression can suggest a change in the speaker or a change in the story's point of view. This feature of ASL body language makes it possible to use a dynamic and captivating storytelling method.

Acquiring proficiency in these nonverbal facets of ASL is equally crucial as learning the signs themselves. They are necessary not just for fluency but also for a more thorough comprehension and admiration of Deaf culture. Understanding these subtleties can assist create connections and friendships outside of the hearing world by fostering bridges with the Deaf community, as ASL is mostly utilized by d/Deaf groups in many nations.

In conclusion, body language and facial expressions in ASL are essential components that give the language grammatical structure, emotional nuance, and clarity. They are not only decorative aspects. Anyone learning ASL has to use them correctly in order to fully integrate into the Deaf community's distinctive cultural and linguistic experience, as well as to communicate efficiently.

CHAPTER 6: HOW TO STRUCTURE A SENTENCE

ASL does not follow English's linear syntax to the letter. Rather, it frequently uses a Topic-Comment framework. With this approach, the signer might first establish the context or subject matter (the topic), then provide more details or a "comment" regarding that topic. Sentence construction can vary depending on the context of the conversation and the relationships between the people speaking due to the flexibility of ASL syntax.

Example: "PIZZA - I LOVE"
- **Topic**: "PIZZA" - Raise your hand in front of you, at shoulder height. Close your fist, leaving only the index and middle fingers extended. With the knuckles of these two fingers slightly bent, move your hand as if you want to draw a 'Z' with the two fingers
- **Comment**: "I LOVE" - Put your finger on your chest to point to yourself ("I"). Then, with each hand in a closed fist, cross your fists over your chest to make the "love" symbol.

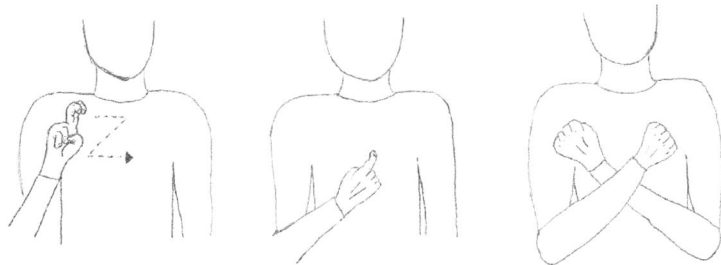

The way that ASL sentences understand time is likewise different from that of English sentences. Time signals in ASL typically begin phrases, providing the temporal context right away. Using "I go to the store tomorrow" as an example would be preferable to "I am going to the store tomorrow."

Example: "Yesterday, we ate pizza"
- **"Yesterday"**: Close your hand into a fist while keeping only your thumb extended. Slide the thumb from the side of your chin down to just below your ear.
- **"We"**: Point towards yourself, then arc your hand inward to include others.

- **"Ate"**: Bring your dominant hand to your mouth as if holding food.
- **"Pizza"**: Hold up your hand shoulder-height in front of you. Only your middle and index fingers should be extending when you close your fist. Move your hand as though you wish to create a 'Z' with these two fingers, with their knuckles slightly bent.

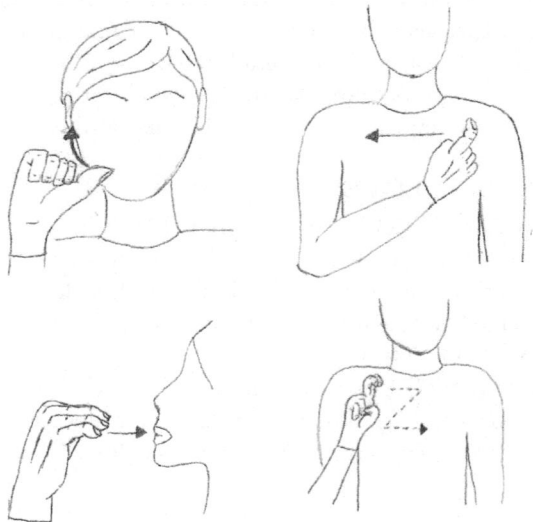

Classifiers, or handshapes that indicate groups or classes of things, people, or ideas, are also used in ASL. These classifiers are used in sentences to characterize the subject's appearance, orientation, movement, and position. For instance, a particular classifier might stand in for a car, and the hand's movements could represent the car's motion.

Example: "A person walking"
- **Classifier for person**: Use your index finger (representing a person).
- **Movement**: "Walk" the finger by alternately tapping the tip of the index finger and the middle finger, moving forward to represent walking.

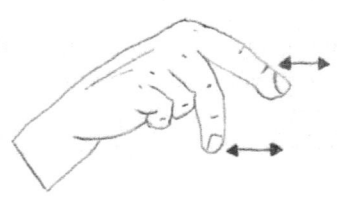

Additionally, ASL utilizes the area surrounding the signer. This spatial component is used to communicate interactions between subjects and objects in a discourse, to depict real or abstract locations, and to indicate various subjects and objects. In order to create both visual and spatial continuity across a discourse, signers can choose a spot in space to represent a person or object and then make references to that space again.

In ASL, the negation is conveyed by non-manual signals like shaking the head or by specialized signs like NOT or NONE. In contrast, negation is frequently incorporated into the verb structure in English.

Example: "I do not understand"
- **Sign for 'I':** Put your finger on your chest to point to yourself
- **Sign for 'Not Understand'**: Raise your fist above your shoulder, with the palm facing towards you, and start shaking your head. Lift your index finger while continuing to shake your head.

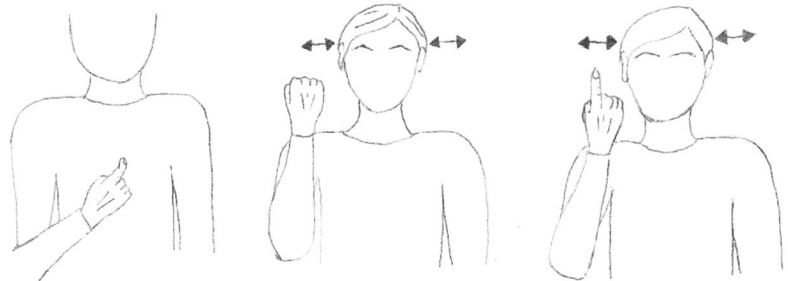

It takes more than just learning the signs to comprehend these nuances of ASL; one must also become fully immersed in the language's distinct structure and cultural setting. It entails a change in perspective from spoken language patterns that are linear to a more spatial and visually focused style of communication. Given how deeply ingrained ASL is in the experiences and worldview of the Deaf community, this change is both linguistic and cultural.

Learners can greatly improve their proficiency by practicing with native signers, interacting with Deaf culture, and using ASL consistently in a variety of settings. These encounters enhance one's comprehension of the grammatical structures as well as one's appreciation of the rich cultural legacy of ASL.

In closing, learning ASL sentence construction involves adjusting to a new, spatially and visually oriented linguistic framework. It entails being aware of the grammar, the significance of non-manual markers, and the cultural background that influences the development of this particular language. For students, frequent practice in authentic environments and proactive involvement with the Deaf community enhance this journey.

CHAPTER 7: MASTERY OF THE ASL ALPHABET: A VISUAL GUIDE

One of the first and most important tasks in learning American Sign Language (ASL) is being proficient in the ASL alphabet. ASL, which is well-known for its expressiveness and visual richness, forms its own alphabet with hand gestures and shapes. Every letter functions as a fundamental instrument for spelling out names, locations, and foreign words as well as a conduit for communication, spanning the gap between silent and expression.

It is important that you practice each letter carefully as you work your way through the ASL alphabet visual guide, paying close attention to the small aspects of hand position, orientation, and movement. Recall that practicing consistently is essential to becoming fluent in ASL. Your ability to spell and comprehend words in ASL will greatly increase as you become more comfortable with each letter. Gaining proficiency in the alphabet is a crucial first step towards becoming skilled in ASL, which can lead to new opportunities for communication and interaction with the deaf and hard-of-hearing community.

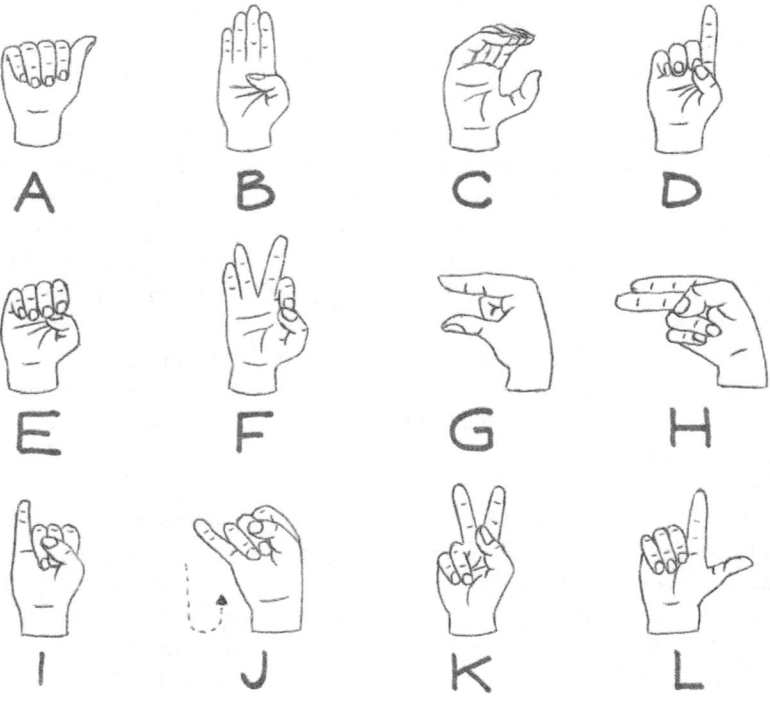

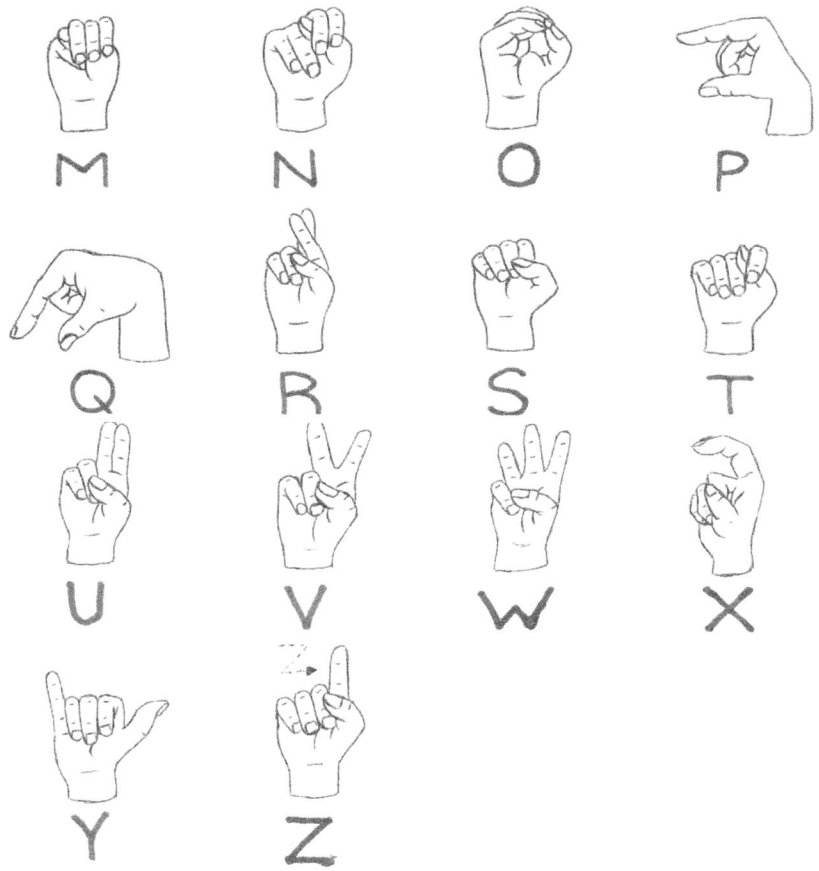

CHAPTER 8: LEARNING NUMBERS IN ASL

In ASL, numbers are more than just hand gestures; they're a smooth fusion of expression and simplicity. Beginners can learn the ins and outs of ASL numbers in this chapter, which covers everything from the fundamentals of one to ten to more intricate formations.

Every ASL number has a distinct handshape and movement that visually conveys its meaning. Acquiring knowledge of these figures involves more than simply learning hand locations; it also entails comprehending how these forms efficiently convey numerical data. This information is essential for everyday conversations as well as more practical ones, such as discussing costs, schedules, or amounts.

This chapter's visual aids will give each number a succinct and understandable portrayal, enabling students to practice and understand these signs. In addition to these illustrations, we will also explore how to place and move your hands to ensure accuracy and clarity when signing numbers.

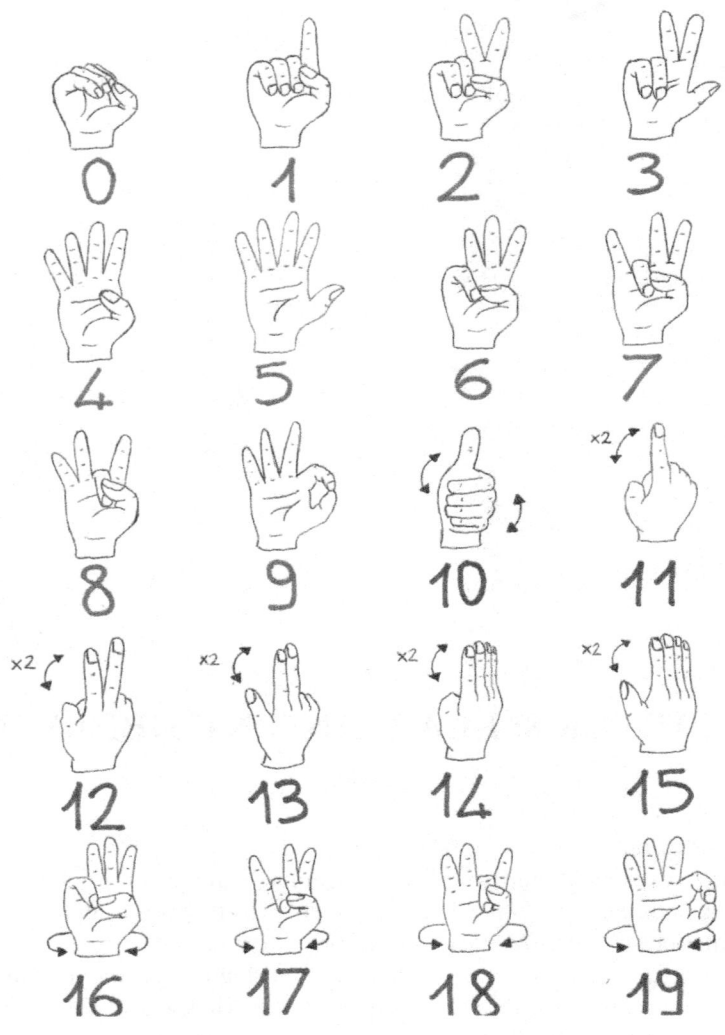

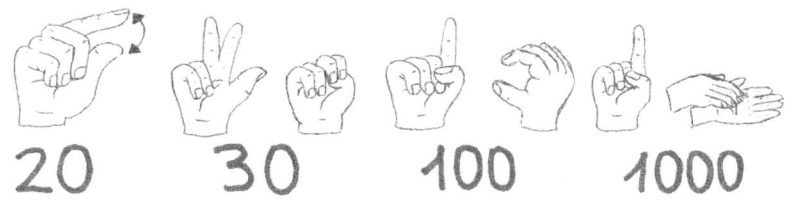

CHAPTER 9: PRACTICAL EXERCISES: SPELLING WORDS AND NUMBERS

Welcome to the area of your ASL learning journey dedicated to practical activities. This chapter intends to give you a set of practical activities to help you hone your ASL fingerspelling and numeracy abilities.

1. Daily Name Challenge: Choose five new names (of persons or places) and fingerspell them every day. As you go, start with shorter names and progressively lengthen and complicate them.

2. Number of the Day: Every day, choose a random number between one and more digits, and practice signing it. Include this figure in several scenarios involving money, time, or quantity.

3. Word Repetition Exercise: Pick a common object and fingerspell its name multiple times during the day, attempting to get faster each time without sacrificing legibility.

4. ASL Number Storytelling: Write numerical stories in quick order. For example, "3 cats watched 2 birds at 1 window," and indicate the numbers in relation to the narrative.

5. Fingerspelling Bee: Finger spelling in the style of a classic spelling bee. One person can fingerspell a word and the others can guess what they think is being spelled. You can work on this with a companion or in a group.

6. Flashcard Practice: Make flashcards by writing the ASL sign for each number on one side and the number on the other. Test yourself frequently or apply them in a gaming environment.

7. Sign Your Day: Try fingerspelling the most important things you did or saw each day, like "coffee," "meeting," "three emails," etc., at the end of the day.

8. ASL Number Puzzles: Make or solve ASL puzzles using numbers, such as basic math problems or sequences, and sign each number as you go.

9. Fingerspelling Memory Game: Try to memorize and sign the complete string of words in the correct order by fingerspelling one word, then adding another to the sequence.

10. Timed Challenge: See how many words or numbers you can successfully fingerspell in a specific amount of time by setting a timer. Monitor your development over time.

You will improve your ability to communicate in ASL more effectively by doing these exercises. Keep in mind that regular practice and real-world application of these skills are the keys to learning fingerspelling and numbers.

BOOK 2: BASIC CONVERSATIONS IN ASL CHAPTER 1: ESSENTIAL SIGNS FOR DAILY COMMUNICATION

A crucial first step in learning American Sign Language (ASL) is becoming proficient in the fundamental vocabulary needed for everyday conversation. This chapter explores the fundamental signs that underpin daily ASL interactions and lay the groundwork for productive and insightful conversations.

1. Child: The sign for "child" involves a simple gesture where you place your open, flat hand at the height of a child's head and then gently pat the air, as if patting the head of a child.

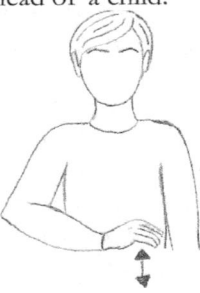

2. Man/Woman: Put your open hand on your forehead and bring it down to your chest to indicate "man." For "woman," in a similar manner, place your open hand close to your chin and bring it down to your chest.

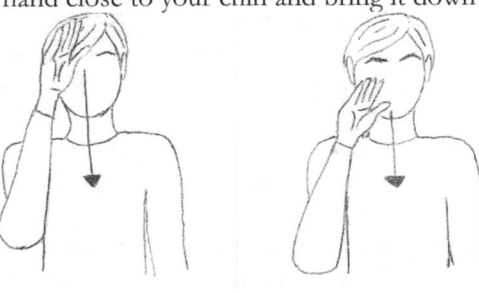

3. What/When/Where/Who/Why/How: These question words are integral to forming inquiries in ASL. Each word has its unique sign:
- **"What"** is signed by holding both hands out, palms up, shrugging your shoulders, and shaking your hands.

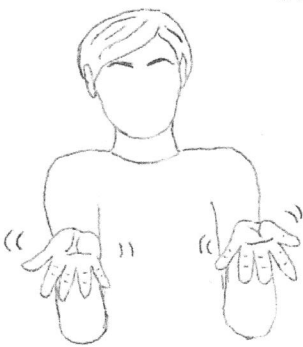

- **"When"** involves making a circular motion with your dominant hand's index finger touching the index finger of your other hand.

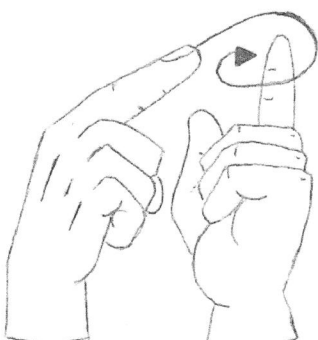

- **"Where"** is signed with an INDEX-finger handshape.

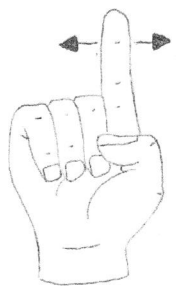

19

- **"Who"** is signed by making the ASL letter "L" with your dominant hand, touching your chin with your thumb, and furrowing your brow while wriggling the longer "L" leg up and down.

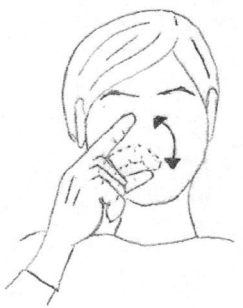

- **"Why"** is formed by placing the fingers of your dominant hand close to your forehead, then moving it forward and downward to form the letter "y," maintaining your palm facing you.

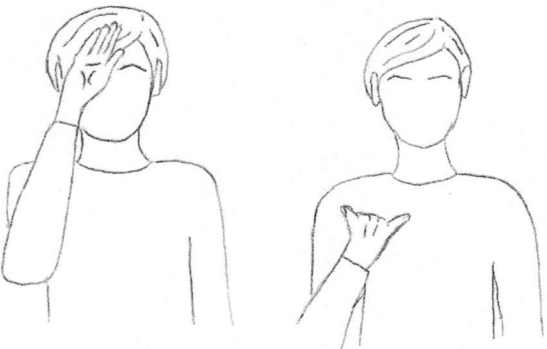

- **"How"** is conveyed using both hands. Create curving forms that are marginally wider than a fist. Rotate your hands 180 degrees while bringing them together such that the knuckles touch.

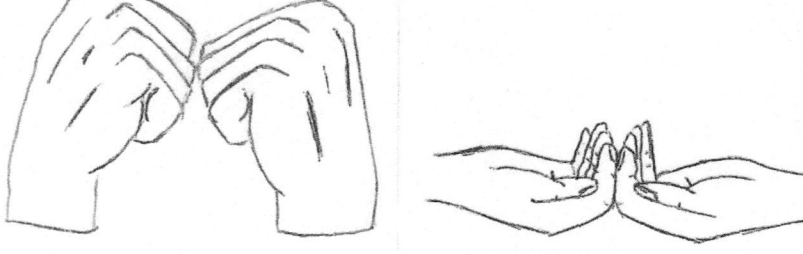

4. Food/Hunger: When you sign "food," picture yourself placing food in your mouth. You may represent "Hunger" by twisting your hand around your stomach in a C shape.

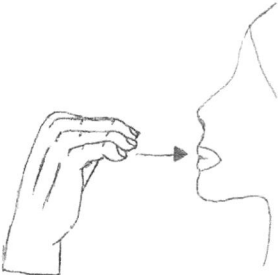

5. Bathroom: The sign for "bathroom" is represented by shaking a "T"-shaped hand.

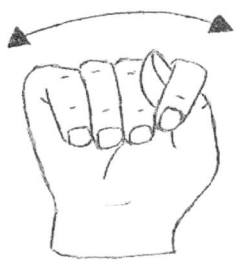

6. Water: To make the "water" sign, shape your right hand into the letter "W." Make two touches with the index finger to the mouth.

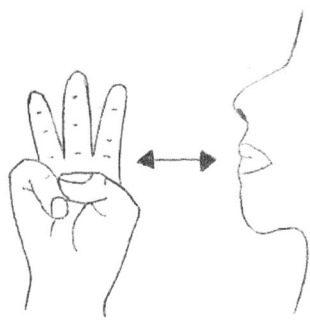

7. Thank You: To show thanks, place a flat palm on your chin and slide it away from your face in a motion similar to blowing a kiss.

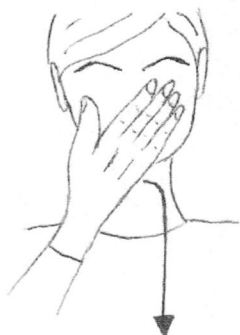

8. School: Clap your open hand like you would if you were hitting a book against your palm, against your non-dominant 'S' hand.

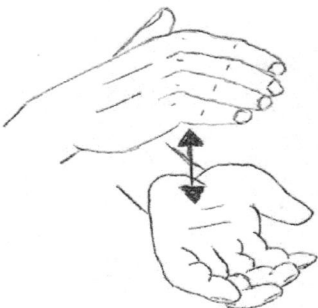

9. Home: Touch your cheek, then your ear, using your index and thumb to symbolize a haven of solace and hearing.

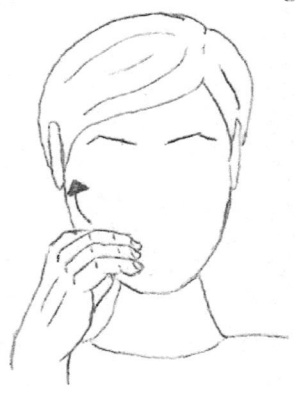

10. Work: Simulate hammering with a fist, which is a common indicator of work.

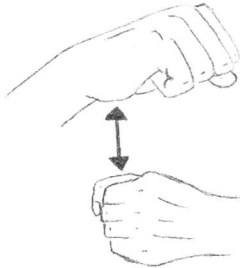

11. Friend: Make a bond by connecting your index fingers. Flip the hands and repeat the same motion.

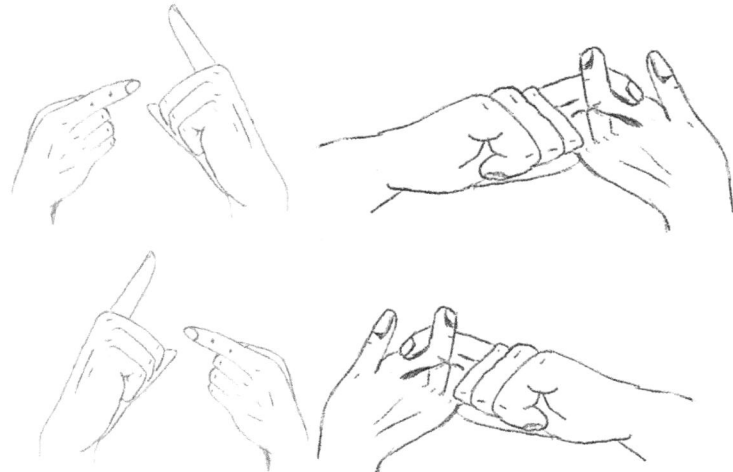

12. Family: Open your hands with the palms facing outward. Join your thumb and index finger, and in this position, rotate your hands in a circular motion so that the palms end up facing inward.

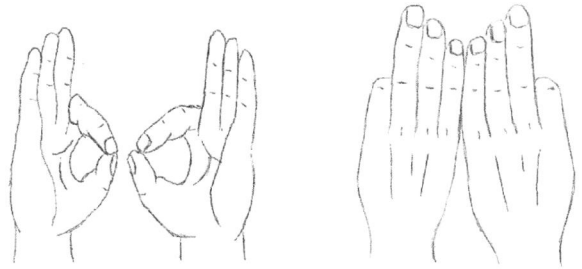

13. Smile: Make a smile appear on your face by using your fingers.

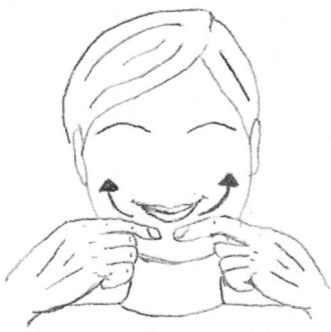

14. Laugh: When you communicate "laugh," add an upward motion to convey happiness.

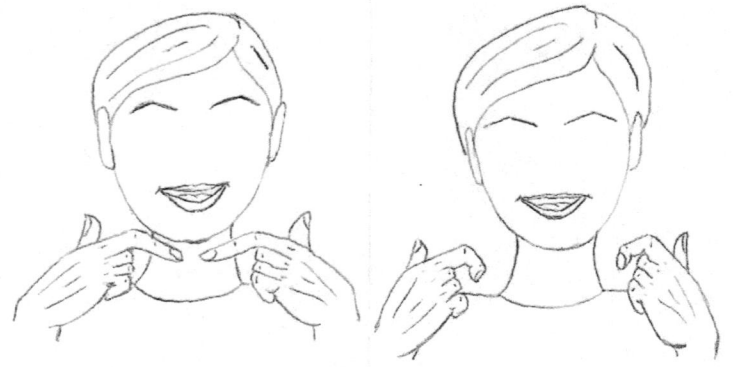

15. Angry: Making "claw" hands and pressing your fingertips to your stomach is how you signify "angry". With both hands, firmly pull up and out.

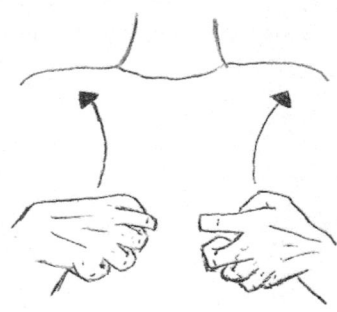

16. Sad: "Sad" is expressed by tracing your fingers across your face in a motion similar to crying.

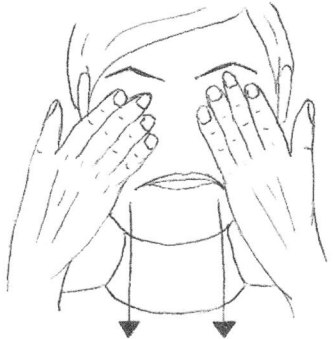

17. Play: Make a 'Y' shape with your hands and shake them to convey a lively motion.

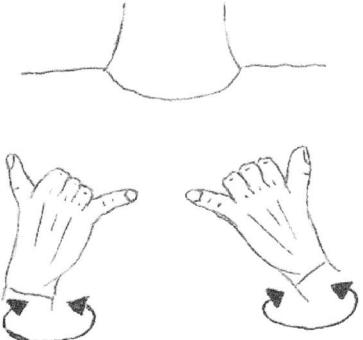

18. Book: Spread your hands wide, like you would when you open a book - a simple metaphor for reading.

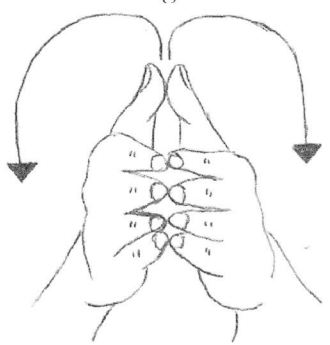

19. Phone: To indicate "phone," simulate to hold a phone up to your ear.

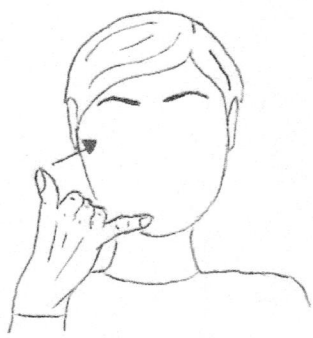

20. Computer: Using the base hand's palm down, the dominant "C" hand circles across its forearm or wrist. Brushing against the back of the base hand is the dominant hand's thumb.

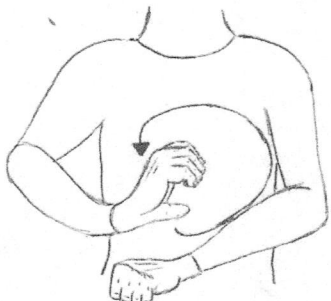

21. Bus/Car: Simply spell B-U-S (very rapidly) to indicate bus. "Car" requires you to imitate a steering wheel utilizing your hands.

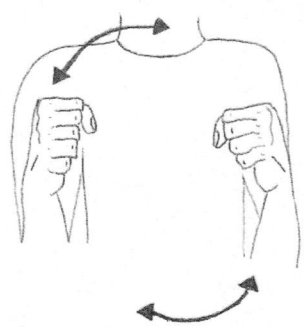

Practical Exercise: ASL Scenarios

Use the signals you've learned to construct brief scenarios or stories to help you remember these important indicators. Write a brief story, for instance, about a typical day in your life using the indicators "home," "work," "food," and "friend." Make advantage of your facial expressions and body language to add more emotion and meaning to your story. Not only will this activity help you practice the signs, but it will also help you become a more proficient ASL communicator. Aim for a minimum of five distinct signs in your narrative, and don't forget to concentrate on the grace notes and legibility of each sign. By using ASL often, you'll become more at ease speaking the language and lay a strong basis for having more intricate conversations.

CHAPTER 2: INTRODUCING YOURSELF AND MAKING CONVERSATION

The essence of human connection is conversations, and in American Sign Language (ASL), this process is expressed precisely and artistically. The goal of this chapter is to help newcomers navigate the subtleties of ASL conversation and introductions, a process that can lead to meaningful personal connections and rich cultural exchanges within the Deaf community.

It is not enough to just translate an English sentence word for word when introducing oneself in ASL. It's about expressing who you are not only with signs but also with body language and facial expressions, which are essential components of ASL grammar. It's usual to introduce oneself and share a little bit of your background with new people you meet.

1. Signing Your Name: Learn to spell your name with your fingers first. Remember that practice makes perfect fingerspelling. For clarity, visualize each letter while maintaining a firm hand position in front of your shoulder.

2. Stating Your Connection to ASL: It's crucial to include information about your affiliation with the ASL community in your introduction. This could entail stating if you are Deaf, hard of hearing people or CODAs (Child of Deaf Adults). Every category has a distinct sign of its own.

- For example, the 'Deaf' sign is indicated by pressing the tip of your index finger to your ear, and then your mouth.

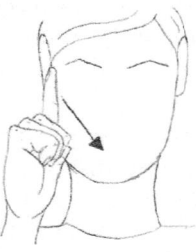

- For "hard to hearing", form a "H" with your hands, drop it a short distance, and watch it bounce up, over, and to the right, then back down in a tiny arc.

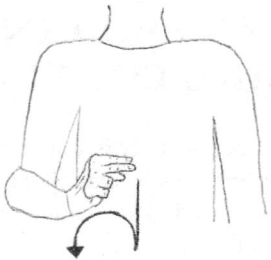

- You would use your fingers to form the letters C-O-D-A if you're a CODA.

These subtleties are important because they let the other person know right away what your background is and foster a closer relationship.

3. Sharing Interests: An interesting method to spice up a discussion is to share your interests or hobbies. Use particular signals to indicate shared interests, such as:

- **Music**: Position your non-dominant forearm across your torso. Next, raise your dominant hand above your other forearm and wave it back and forth like you're leading an orchestra.

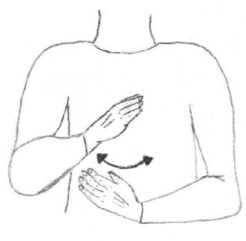

- **Art**: Raise the hand that is not your dominant in opposite you, palm regarding your visage, to sign "art." With the pinky finger of your dominant hand, make a zig-zag motion as if to simulate that you are painting.

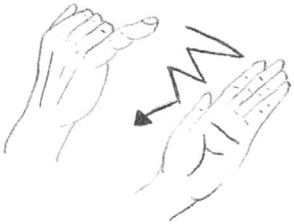

- **Sports**:
  Basketball: Rotate your hands back and forth, holding them as though you were holding a basketball.

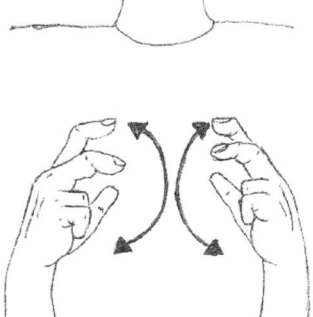

Baseball: Liken it to a baseball bat swing.

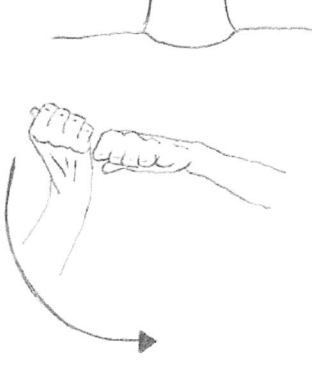

Football: Interlock and unlock your fingers repeatedly.

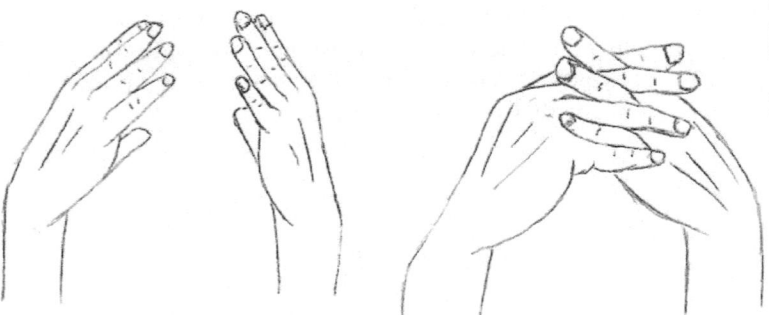

Reading: Using your dominant hand, which stands for eyes, make a 'V' and run it along your open palm, which represents a page.

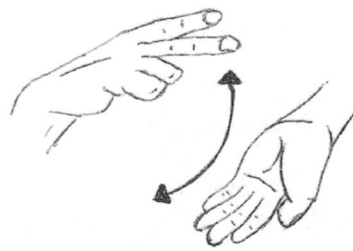

Cooking: Simulate flipping pancakes, hold the skillet flat with one hand and flip with the other.

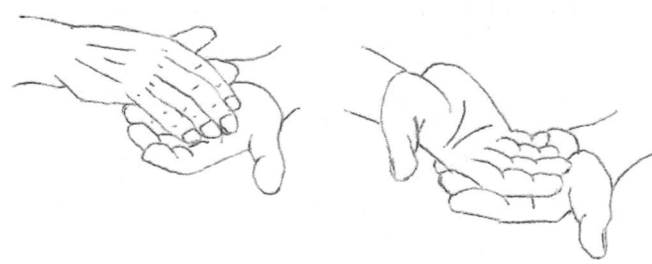

    4. Asking Questions: Expressing interest in the other person is a prerequisite for starting a discussion. Make use of open-ended inquiries to get more detailed answers. Recall that while asking questions in ASL, people frequently lift their eyebrows for yes/no questions and furrow them for WH queries (who, what, where, when, and why).
    5. Understanding Turn-Taking: Like a dance, ASL talks have a

rhythm. Remember to listen and to acknowledge when it is your moment to talk. Important indicators that demonstrate you are following along are nodding and keeping eye contact.

6. Expressing Emotions: Facial expressions in ASL are a rich way to convey emotions. Each emotion changes its representation to reflect the intensity of feeling, whether it be happiness, sadness, surprise, or fury. Your signs can have a very different meaning when you smile or grimace.

7. Closing the Conversation: Use suitable farewell signs such as "GOODBYE," "SEE YOU LATER," or "NICE TO MEET YOU" when it's time to part ways. These not only indicate the conclusion of the discussion but also make a positive impact.

Practice Exercise: Introduce Yourself in ASL

1. Record a video of yourself introducing yourself in ASL. Make sure your fingers are moving smoothly and clearly as you begin by fingerspelling your name.

2. Indicate in the same video how you are connected to the ASL community, regardless of whether you are hearing people studying ASL or Deaf, hard of hearing, or a CODA. Don't forget to use the right indication for each category.

3. Make use of specific ASL signs to share two of your hobbies.

4. Ask a brief closing question at the end of your introduction, such as "What about you?" Always remember to modify your expressions to fit the kind of question you are posing.

5. Finally, end with a sign such as 'GOODBYE' or 'NICE TO MEET YOU'.

Examine your video once it has been recorded. Take note of the way you flow from one section of your introduction to the next, the clarity of your signs, and your facial emotions. You'll feel more at ease introducing yourself and having simple ASL discussions if you do this activity.

CHAPTER 3: GREETINGS, FAREWELLS, AND EVERYDAY PHRASES

For newcomers, learning basic greetings, goodbyes, and phrases in American Sign Language (ASL) is crucial since it establishes the basis for everyday communication. Connecting with the Deaf population and having basic conversations is made possible by these basic signs.

1. Greetings:
- **Hello**: With your hand resting on your temple and the palm facing forward, extend your hand and gently move it from side to side.

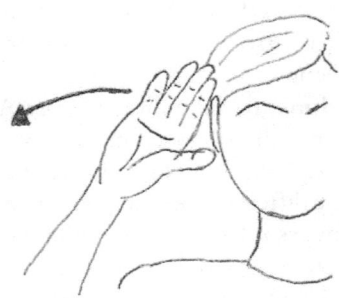

- **Good Morning**: Even though we often use two hands to sign "morning," we frequently only use one hand to say ordinary phrases like "Good morning." When signing GOOD-MORNING while holding a cup of hot chocolate, the one-handed variation comes in handy. To sign "good morning," rest your open hand under your lip and then extend your arm forward while keeping your elbow close to your body.

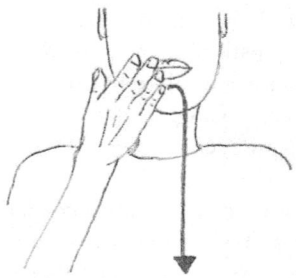

- **Good Afternoon**: For 'good' rest your open hand under your lip. Simply point ahead and slightly up with your dominant flat hand to make the "afternoon" sign.

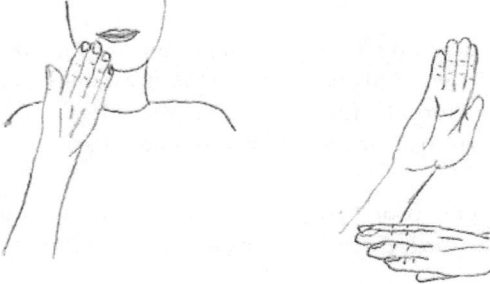

- **Good Evening**: Sign 'good' as before. To make the "evening" sign, hold your non-dominant arm horizontally and point to the side with the palm down. Place the wrist of your dominant hand, fingertips down, on the back of your non-dominant hand.

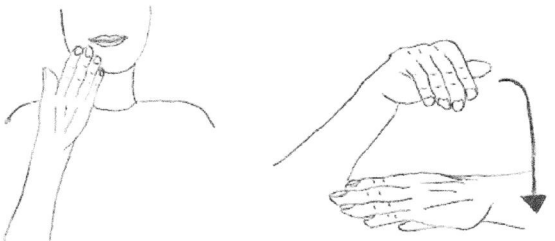

2. **Farewells**:
    - **Goodbye**: Fold your fingers down and open your palm, then do it again.

    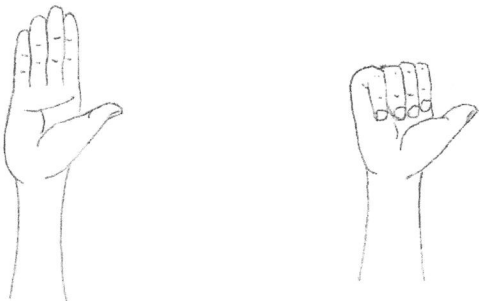

    - **See You Later**: Sign 'see' by pointing to your eyes, then 'later' by making the "Future" sign with an "L" handshape.

    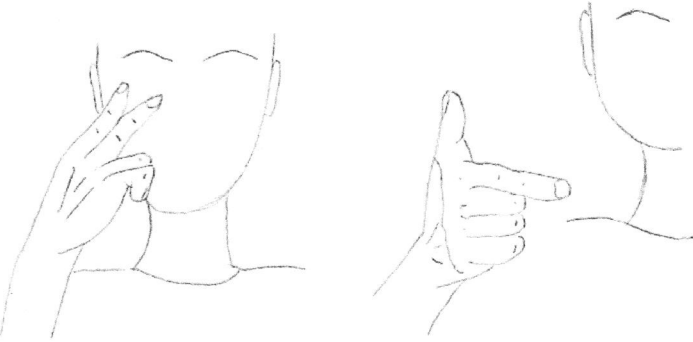

- **Take Care**: Twice, the left "K" hand is struck by the right "K" hand. Though the left hand moves a little as well, the right hand does the most of the work:

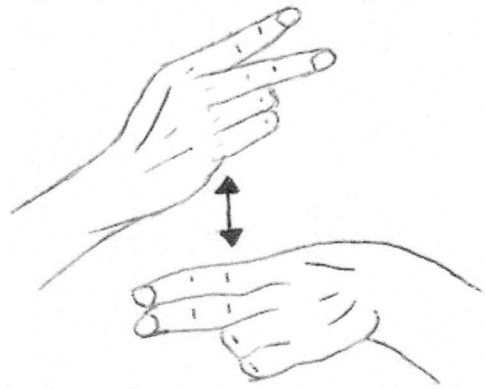

3. **Everyday Phrases**:
   - **Sorry**: Create a circle around your heart.

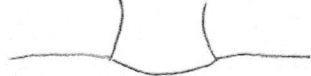

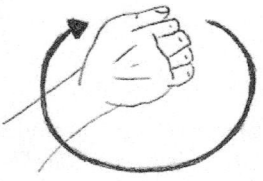

- **Yes**: Close your hand into a fist. While keeping your arm still, bend the fist up and down at the wrist, as if nodding.

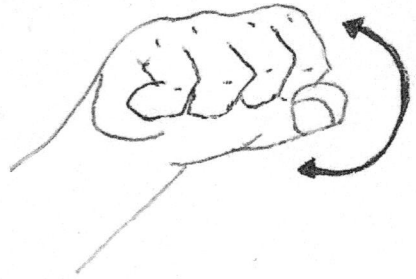

- **No**: With your hand open, bring your index and middle fingers to meet your thumb, opening and closing them several times. You can also accompany this gesture with a head shake for "no."

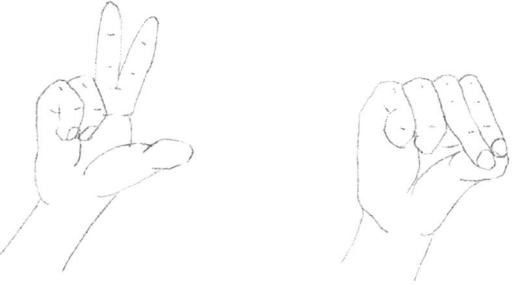

- **Please**: Make a circular motion with your flat hand on your chest.

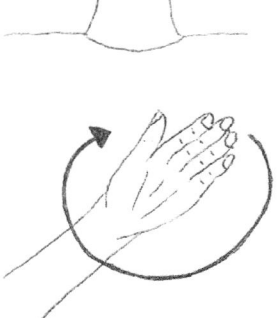

- **Excuse Me**: With the palm of your non-dominant hand facing the sky, run the fingertips of your dominant hand over your palm many time.

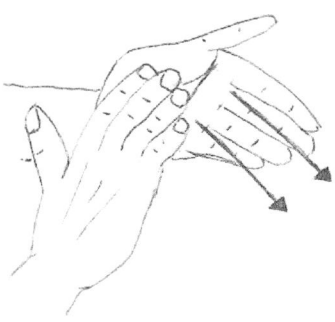

- **Help**: Close one hand into a fist but with the thumb raised, and rest it on your other open hand with the palm facing up. While maintaining this position, slowly lift both hands together upwards.

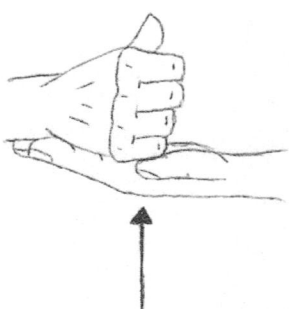

- **Where is the bathroom?**: "Where" is signed with an INDEX-finger handshape. The sign for "bathroom" is represented by shaking a "T"-shaped hand.

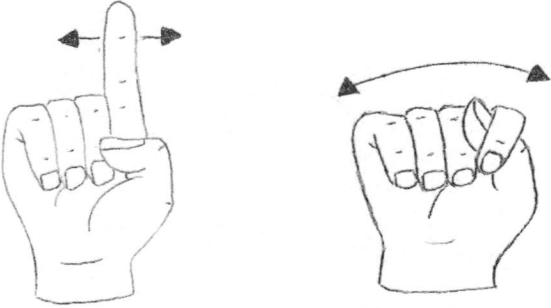

- **I like**: Start by signing "I" by pointing to yourself. Then touch your chest with an open hand, and as you move it away, sign the number "8."

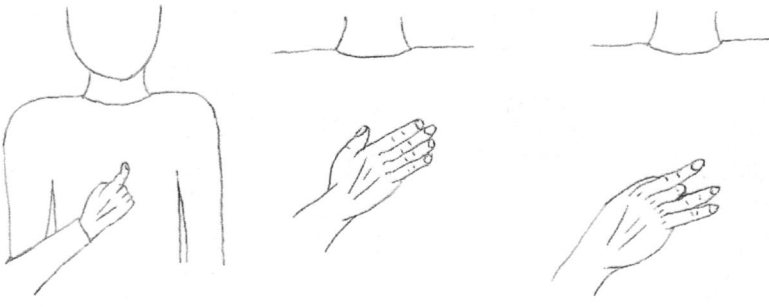

- **I love**: Sign "I" first, pointing to yourself. Then, with each hand in a closed fist, cross your fists over your chest to make the "love" symbol.

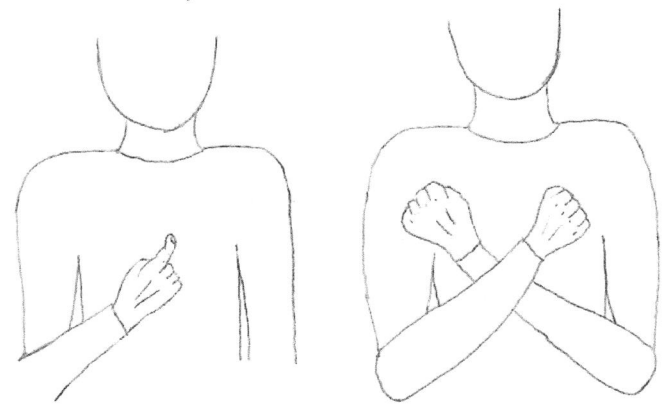

- **I hate**: First, sign "I" and point to yourself. Then sign "8" with both hands and open them completely.

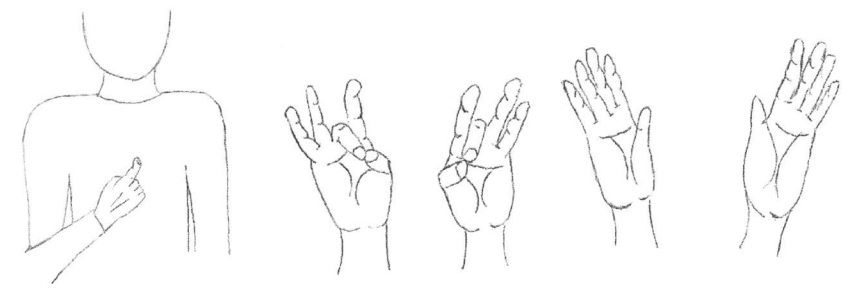

- **Repeat**: Open your non-dominant hand completely and partially open your dominant hand. Touch the fingers of your dominant hand to the palm of your other hand.

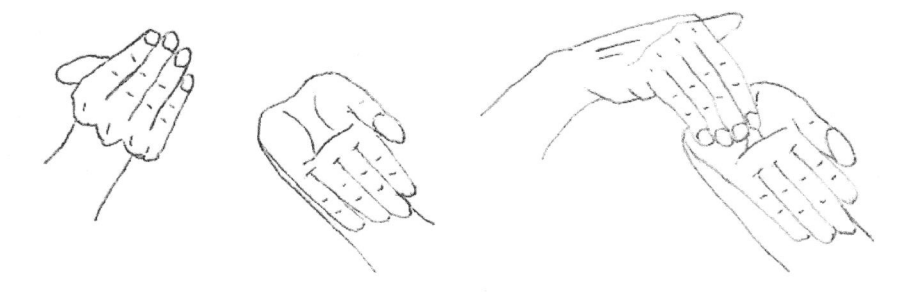

4. Basic Questions:
- **How are you?**: Start with "How": Make curved shapes that are just a little bit larger than a fist. Bring your hands together until the knuckles meet, then turn them 180 degrees. Then point to the other person for "YOU."

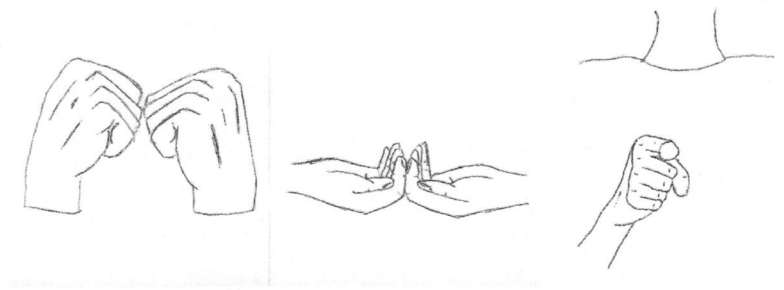

- **What's your name?**: First, open your hand in front of you and sign "your" with the palm looking outward. Then sign "name" by closing both hands into fists, keeping only the index and middle fingers extended. Once in this position, tap the open fingers of your dominant hand against the non-dominant hand several times. Conclude with "what" by holding both hands out, palms up, shrugging your shoulders, and shaking your hands.

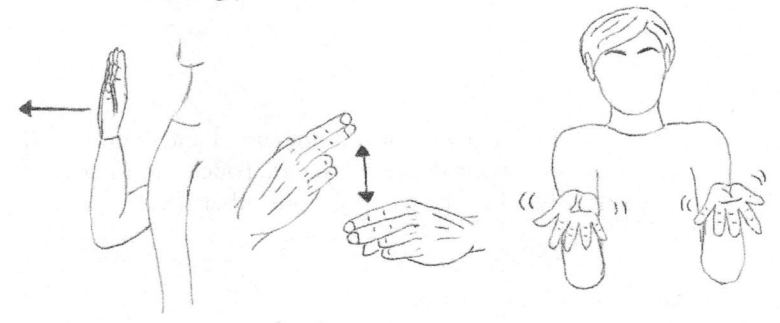

- **Where are you from?**: Point to the other person for "YOU." Pull your dominant hand away from your non-dominant hand as if you were pulling back a string on a bow. "Where" is signed with an INDEX-finger handshape.

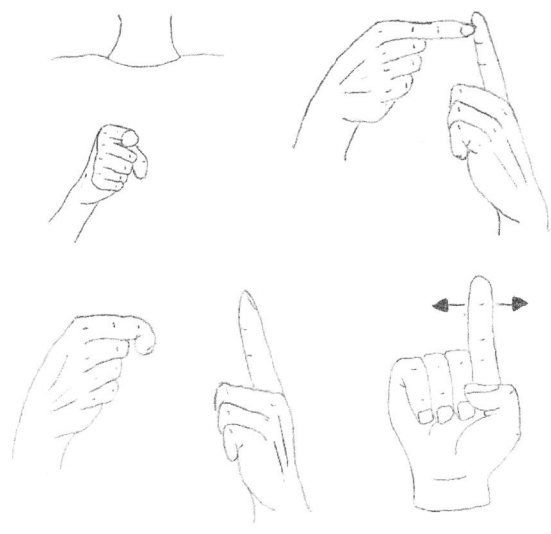

- **Are you deaf?**: The "ARE" sign is often not regarded as ASL. It is usually able to be dropped. 'Deaf' sign is indicated by pressing the tip of your index finger to your ear, and then your mouth. To finish, point to the other person to sign 'YOU.'

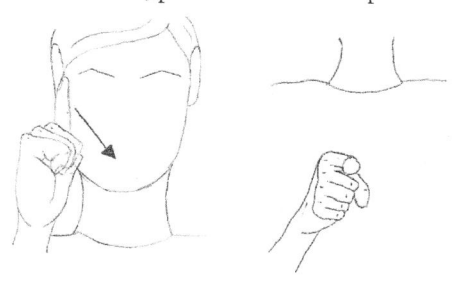

- **How old are you?**: Point at the other person to sign "YOU" to begin. Sign 'old' by pulling the imaginary beard down from your chin many time.

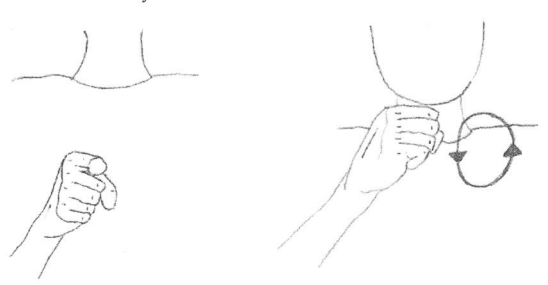

- **Do you have siblings?**: Start by signing "siblings" by opening both hands into an "L" shape. With your dominant hand, start from your forehead and, maintaining the "L" shape, bounce it twice on your non-dominant hand. Continue by pointing for "YOU." Conclude by bringing both hands, slightly bent, to your chest to sign "HAVE."

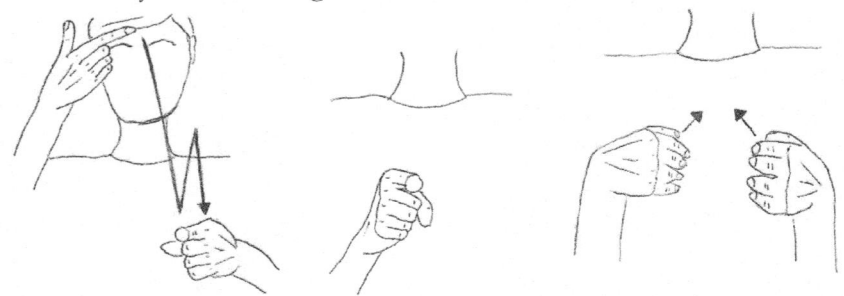

Practice Exercise

Readers are asked to practice regularly as a practical exercise to help them absorb these ideas. Every day, set aside 10 to 15 minutes to practice these hellos, goodbyes, and common phrases in front of a mirror. Begin by signing each word slowly, paying attention to the correctness of your hand movements and shapes. As you become more comfortable, steadily increase your speed. Make a video of yourself signing these sentences as well. Watch the video again to evaluate your own skill level and pinpoint areas that need work. This practice improves confidence in using ASL for basic communication while also strengthening muscle memory. Recall that the secret to acquiring these fundamental ASL skills is constant practice.

CHAPTER 4: SIGNS FOR FAMILY MEMBERS AND RELATIONSHIPS

In the fields of American Sign Language (ASL), family and relationship communication is an essential component of daily interactions. This chapter explores the signs for different family members and connections and offers a detailed explanation on how to use each sign appropriately.

- **Mother**

Handshape: Open palm with fingers spread apart.
Movement: Place your open hand by your chin and tap it twice.

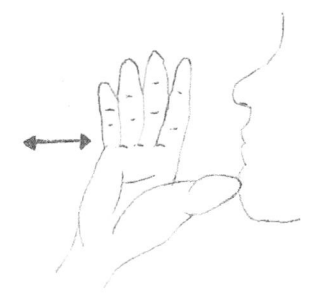

- **Father**

Handshape: Same as 'Mother.'
Movement: Similar to 'Mother,' but the hand starts from the forehead, not the chin.

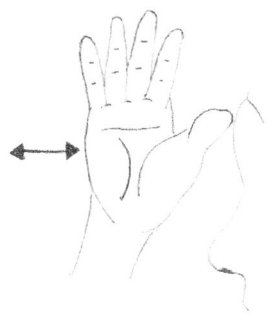

- **Brother**

Handshape: Start with an 'L' shape (index and thumb extended).
Movement: Open both hands into an "L" shape. The dominant hand should start from the forehead and touch the non-dominant hand only once.

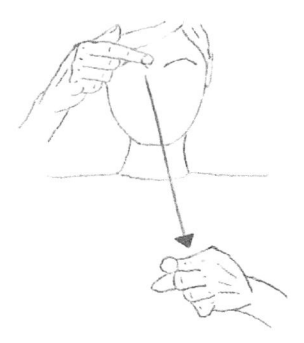

- **Sister**

Handshape: Begin with the 'L' shape.

Movement: Open both hands into an "L" shape. The dominant hand should start from the chin and touch the non-dominant hand only once.

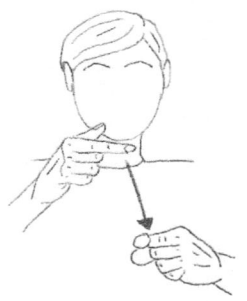

- **Son**

Handshape: Start with a flat hand.

Movement: Start with your dominant hand touching your temple and your non-dominant hand bent at waist level. Complete the sign by moving your dominant hand from your head down to rest it on your non-dominant arm.

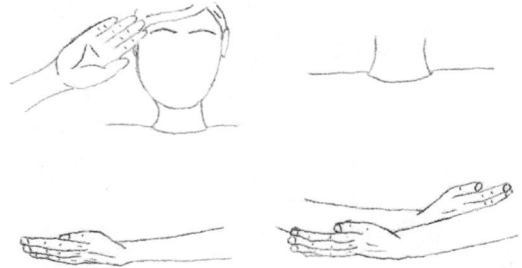

- **Daughter**

Handshape: Begin with a flat hand.

Movement: Start with your dominant hand touching your chin and your non-dominant hand bent at waist level. Complete the sign by moving your dominant hand down to rest it on your non-dominant arm.

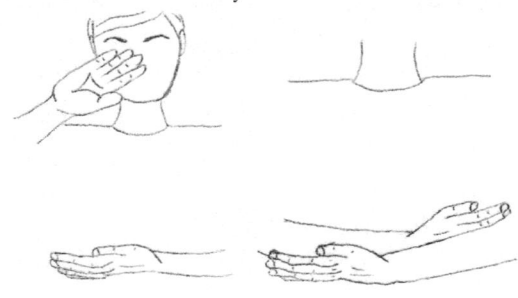

- **Grandparents**

Handshape: Same as 'Mother' and 'Father.'

Movement: For 'Grandfather,' start the 'Father' sign and move it forward in two small arches. Repeat similarly for 'Grandmother,' starting from the chin.

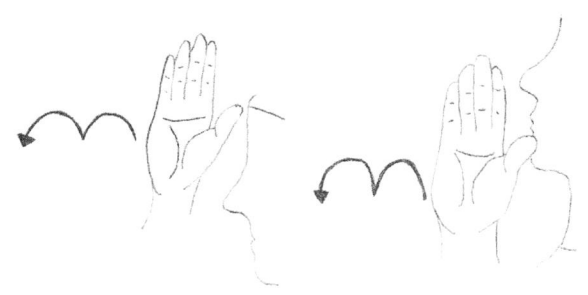

- **Spouse (Husband/Wife)**

Handshape: The dominant hand should be almost completely open, and the non-dominant hand should form a "C" shape.

Movement: Position the dominant hand next to your head. Then, lower the hand and close it onto the other hand in front of you two times, almost as if you are about to clap your hands.

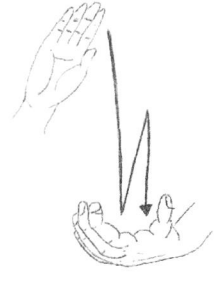

- **Boyfriend**

Handshape: Form your hand into a beak-like shape, with fingers touching the thumb.

Movement: Bring your dominant hand in a beak shape to your forehead, then touch the fingers with the thumb. Finally, sign "friend" by touching the index fingers of both hands together.

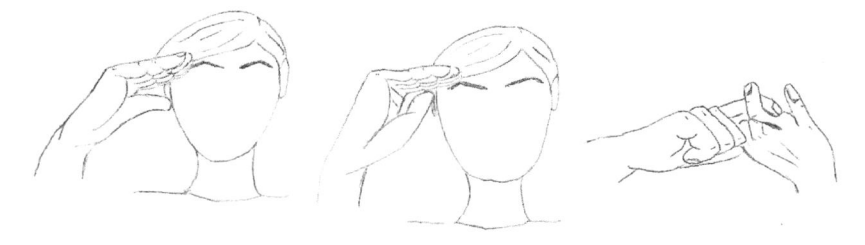

- **Girlfriend**

Handshape: Slide the thumb from the cheek down to the chin.

Movement: Alternate touching the index fingers of each hand, first placing one index finger over the other and then switching, creating an alternating motion between the two index fingers.

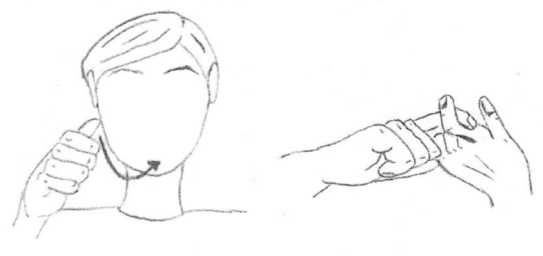

- **Baby**

Handshape: Arms cradle an imaginary baby.

Movement: Rock your arms back and forth as if holding and soothing a baby.

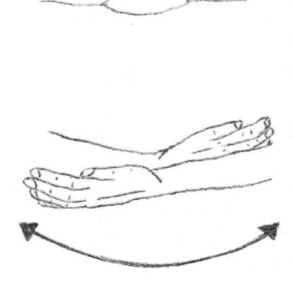

Family Tree Exercise in ASL

Make a visual family tree using the parents, siblings, grandparents, and other family members discussed in this chapter. As you point to each member of your family on your tree, practice signing their title. Introduce each member in ASL first, making use of the particular hand forms and motions you have studied. Say "mother," for instance, and then gesture to her photo on your tree. For each family member, follow these procedures once more.

By linking the signs to particular family members, this activity will help reinforce the signs and improve memory recall and comprehension.

CHAPTER 5: TIME AND DATES IN ASL

In addition to being a useful ability, knowing how to communicate in American Sign Language (ASL) about time and dates can lead to more in-depth discussions about calendars, events, and history. The key signals for expressing time ideas, days of the week, and dates in ASL are covered in this chapter.

Expressing General Time Concepts

- **Now**: Drop the "Y" hands a couple of inches.

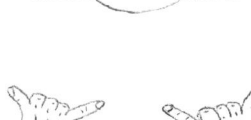

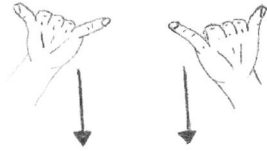

- **Later**: There are a couple of versions to indicate "LATER." The most typical is the one with the forward-facing "L"-shaped hand.

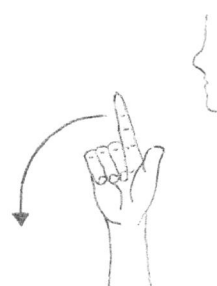

- **Before**: Flick your dominant hand backward over your shoulder, starting with the hand in front of your body.

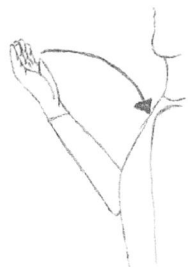

- **Soon**: Perform the action with a hand shaped like the letter "F" and make a double tapping motion near the mouth. Gently tap your chin two times.

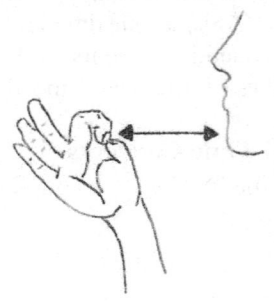

- **Eventually**: With a relaxed hand, make a forward motion.

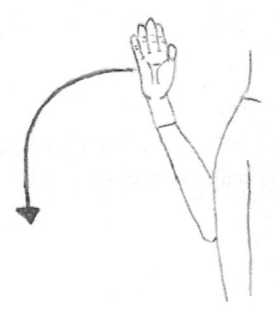

Days of the Week

In this chapter, we explore the days of the week in American Sign Language (ASL). Below, you will find detailed pictures for each day, designed to aid in your visual comprehension and practice of these essential signs. The days are presented in the following order: Sunday, Monday, Tuesday, Wednesday, Thursday, Friday, and Saturday.

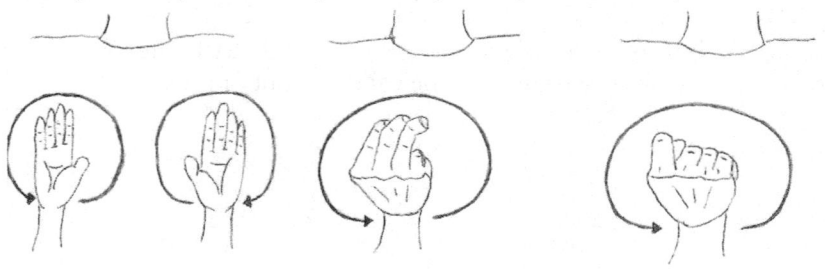

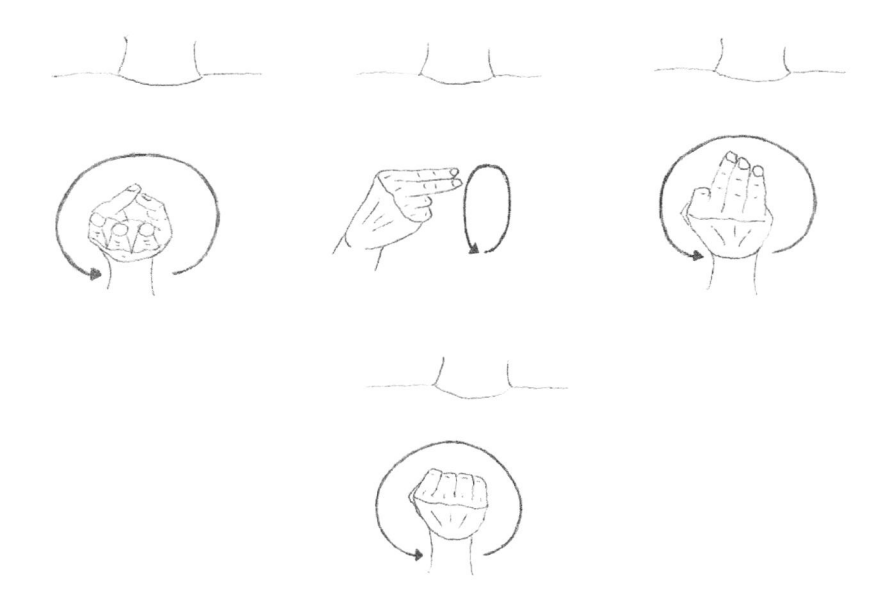

Months

Generally, the months of the year are fingerspelled in ASL. This can be written out whole, as "MARCH," or in shorthand, like "JAN" for January. It's vital to remember that different persons fingerspell the months at different rates; some fingerspell the months rapidly, while others do so more slowly. Improving your comprehension of fast fingerspelling will be essential as you learn ASL, particularly for understanding these calendar phrases.

Combining Dates and Times

Combine the time and date indicators when talking about particular occasions. If the event is scheduled for June 15 at 3 PM, for example, you may write "June" (fingerspell), "15" (number sign), "afternoon" (sun position), and "3" (number sign).

Recall that body language and facial expressions are essential for communicating the subtleties of dates and time in ASL. Making an expressive communicating might assist highlight the urgency or carefree atmosphere of the moment you are talking about.

Practical Exercise for Readers

Here is a useful activity to aid with the assimilation of the concepts discussed in this chapter: Using ASL, make a weekly schedule. Begin by writing the days of the week, then follow each day with particular times and activities. Sign "Monday", "morning", and "baseball" for example. Try this out every day of the week at various times and with different exercises. Observe your body language and facial emotions to convey the type of activity you are doing, whether it is a routine task or something you are looking forward to. This practice will help you become more proficient at integrating several ASL elements to communicate complicated thoughts, as well as strengthen your mastery of time and date signs.

CHAPTER 6: BUILDING VOCABULARY: ADJECTIVES AND ADVERBS IN ASL

Increasing your vocabulary in American Sign Language (ASL) and putting particular emphasis on adjectives and adverbs will help you communicate in vivid detail. This chapter offers a practical method for learning these grammatical constructions. We go into great depth about each sign so you can learn and practice with ease. Keep in mind that your ability to communicate effectively in ASL is influenced by your body language and facial expressions in addition to the signs itself.

List of Common Adjectives and Adverbs
- **Big**: Start with your hands close but not touching, palms facing each other and index fingers slightly bent. Then move them horizontally, as if showing the size of something large.

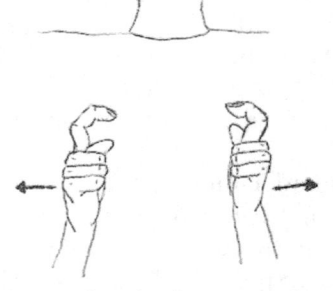

- **Small**: Bring your hands close to each other. This sign imitates the gesture of indicating something very small.

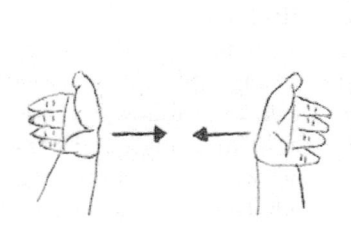

- **Hot**: Bring your hand to your mouth as if you are eating something and then quickly throw it downwards, as if you have been burned.

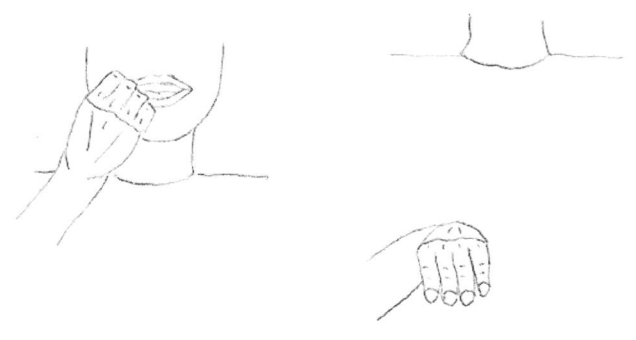

- **Cold**: Raise both of your fists to below shoulder height. Next, repeatedly move your fists in a rhythmic manner toward and away from one another, as though you were feeling chilly.

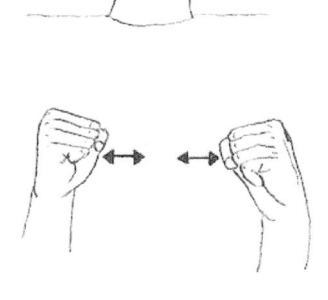

- **Happy**: Smile broadly as you sign, with your hands moving upwards from your chest and then cycling back down. Your facial expression is crucial here.

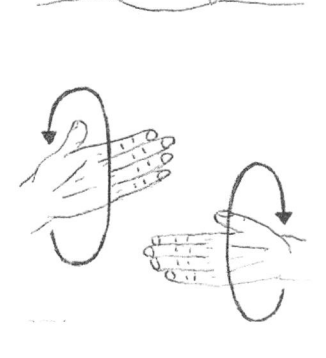

- **Quickly**: Start with both hands in a fist but with the index fingers slightly open. With a swift movement, close the fists completely and open only the thumbs.

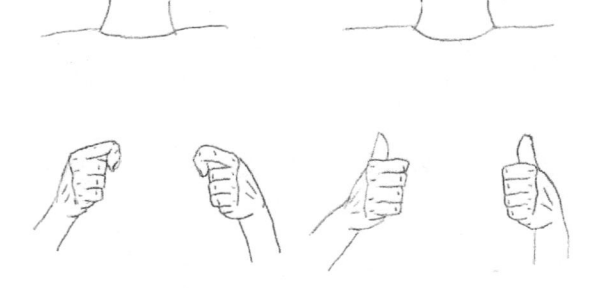

- **Slowly**: For the sign 'slow,' gently slide your dominant hand along the back of your non-dominant hand. Start this motion from the back of the base of the non-dominant hand, moving upwards just a few inches.

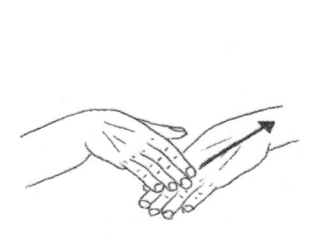

- **Carefully**: "Place your right 'K' hand over your left 'K' hand, assuming you are right-handed. Keep your hands together in this position and without separating them, make a circular movement by moving them forward, then down, back, and up again. Accompany this motion with a facial expression that conveys caution."

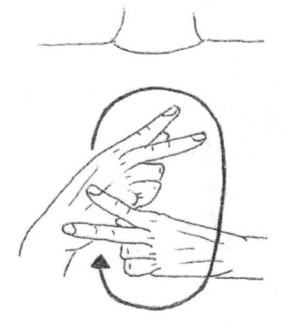

Practical Exercise: Creating Descriptive Sentences in ASL

First, choose three terms from this chapter's lists of adjectives and adverbs. It is your task to construct ASL sentences using the adjectives or adverbs you have selected.

1. Visualize: Think over the sentence before you sign. Consider the situation in which this adverb or adjective would be appropriate.

2. Express: Pay close attention to your body language and facial expressions as you sign each statement. Recall that in ASL, these non-manual cues are essential for expressing the complete meaning of adjectives and adverbs.

3. Record and Review: Make a video of yourself signing these sentences, if you can. When you watch the recordings, focus on how you employ facial expressions, how clearly you sign, and how naturally you communicate overall.

4. Reflect: Consider the experience after you've finished the exercise. Which gestures or facial expressions feel more appropriate? Was it difficult for you to include the non-manual signals?

This practice will help you communicate more effectively and with greater nuance by expanding your vocabulary and developing your expressive ASL skills.

CHAPTER 7: SIGNS FOR COMMON ACTIVITIES AND HOBBIES

This chapter explores how ordinary activities and hobbies might be described using the expressive language of American Sign Language (ASL). ASL facilitates the vibrant exchange of hobbies and interests, making it more than merely a language of need. We go over important indicators for a variety of pastimes here, with enough detail to improve your ASL conversational skills. We will now discuss other hobbies in addition to the ones we just covered in Chapter 2, "Introducing Yourself," which include reading, cooking, music, art, football, baseball, and basketball.

- **Gardening**

Description: This hobby is signed in two stages. The first stage involves representing a plant emerging from the ground using both hands. The second stage signs by simulating digging in a cyclical manner using both hands.

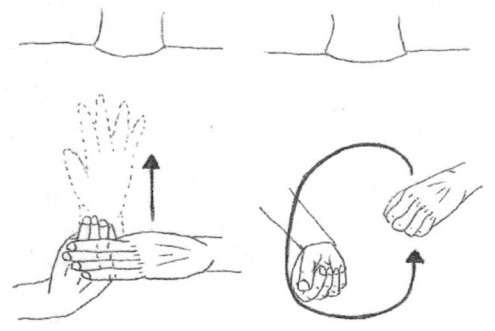

- **Swimming**

Description: Moving forward in unison, both hands imitate a swimming motion.

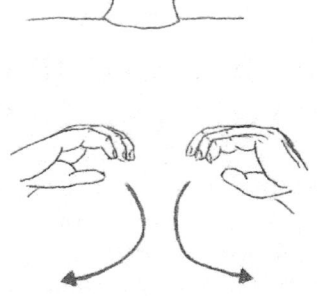

- **Photography**

Description: With both hands, draw a rectangle as though you were framing a picture, then simulate clicking with both indexes.

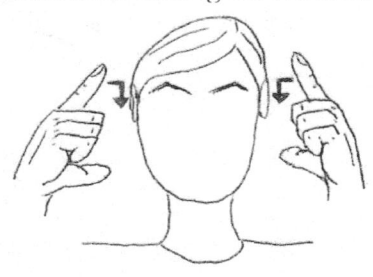

- **Hiking**

Description: Using both hands with the palms facing downwards, mimic a motion that swings alternately from right to left while simultaneously moving forward.

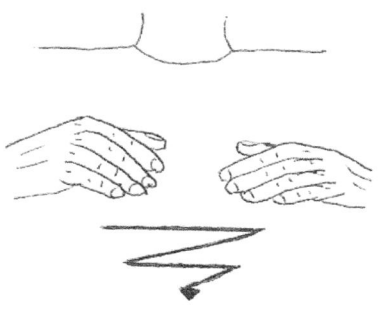

- **Yoga**

Description: In a prayer pose, join your hands in front of your chest. Maintain this position to represent the standard yoga pose.

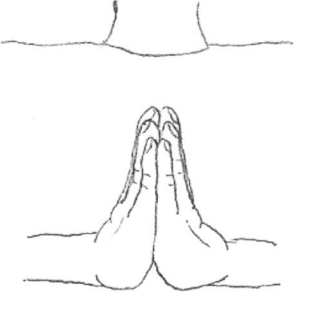

- **Sewing**

Description: With your dominant hand, pretend to hold a needle and make tiny, light sewing motion as though you are threading a needle into fabric.

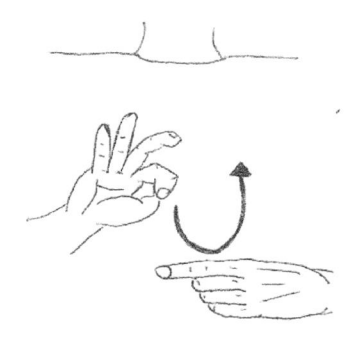

- **Skiing**

Description: Pretending to hold ski poles, keep your index fingers slightly open and make small up and down movements.

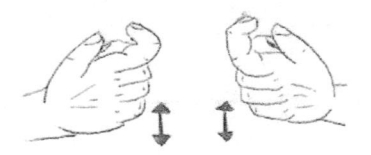

Exercise: Create Your ASL Hobby Story

Using the hobby indications covered in this chapter, write a little story about your favorite activity. Start by using ASL to describe the location (such as a park, your house, or a beach). Next, add three or more of the hobby indications (such gardening, swimming, or photography) that you studied in this chapter. For example, you could write that you go swimming in the afternoon, spend your mornings gardening, and finish the day by taking pictures of the setting sun. Try fluently signing this story, paying attention to how you move between signs and how you incorporate appropriate body language and expressions. This practice helps you learn the signs by heart and enhances your ability to tell stories in ASL that make sense.

CHAPTER 8: FOOD AND BEVERAGES: FROM GROCERY SHOPPING TO DINING OUT

Getting about the food and drink world is a fun part of everyday life, and when done in American Sign Language (ASL), it becomes an interesting means of discussing eating customs, tastes, and culinary adventures. This chapter offers a complete guide to assist you in a variety of culinary situations, with a focus on the practical ASL signs relating to food, beverages, grocery shopping, and dining out.

- **Drink/Beverage**

Description: Bring a cup to your lips in the impression that you are sipping from it.

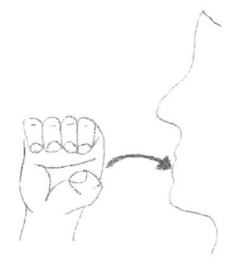

- **Grocery Store**

Description: Start by signing 'food' or 'eat'. Do this by repeatedly touching your fingers to your mouth, indicating the act of eating. Then, proceed with the sign for 'store' by joining your thumbs to the other fingers and shaking your hand outward.

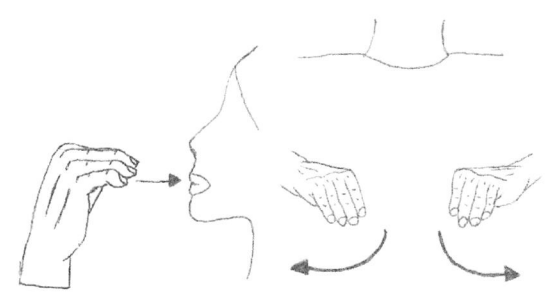

- **Buy/Purchase**

Description: Hold your non-dominant hand slightly tilted and your dominant hand behind it. With a simple movement, move the dominant hand over the non-dominant one, now placing the dominant hand closer to the interlocutor, as if to give money.

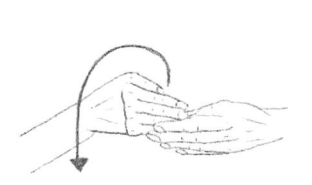

- **Fruit**

Description: Touch the tips of your thumb and index finger to your cheek while forming a "F" hand shape. Twirl the "F"-hand twice over your cheek, maintaining contact as you make the sign. Make sure the hand remains in the same location on your cheek, not slipping or shifting.

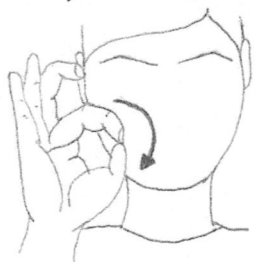

- **Vegetables**

Description: Form the letter 'V' with your hand. Keep the index finger steady on your cheek and rotate the middle finger twice until it touches the chin.

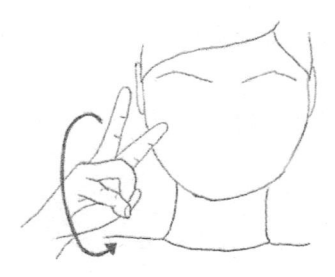

Dining Out Signs
- **Restaurant**

Description: Form a "R" with your hand and place it against one corner of your chin. Next, tap the opposite chin corner with the same hand motion.

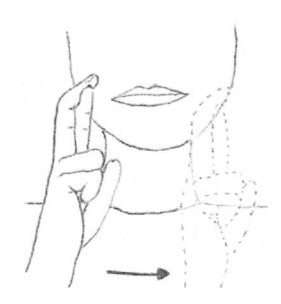

- **Menu**

Description: Start by signing 'food' as seen in previous sections. Then, open your non-dominant hand with the palm facing upwards and with your dominant hand vertical, tap in multiple spots getting closer to the wrist. Finish by signing 'book' as we learned previously.

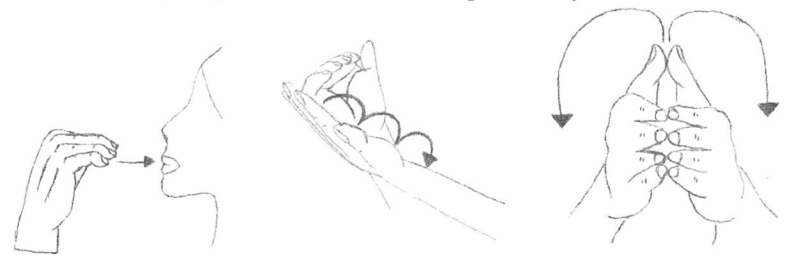

- **Order**

Description: Starting with the index finger of your dominant hand touching your lip, make a forward motion while keeping your wrist steady.

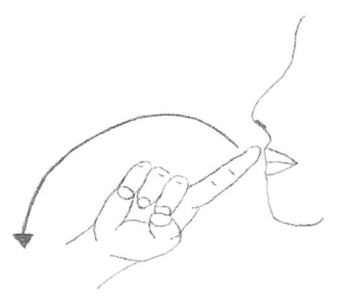

- **Bill/Check**

Description: The most common method for signing this word is through fingerspelling.

- **Tip**

Description: Similar to 'bill,' to sign this word, it is sufficient to finger spell using the alphabet learned in the early chapters.

Practical Exercise

An enjoyable and instructive practical practice can be used to further reinforce the lessons learned in this chapter on food and beverages in ASL. At home, set up a fictitious eating situation. Using the ASL signs you have learnt, start by 'ordering' a dinner. You can even sign the item you would like to order and even ask for a receipt. Using the signals for different food products and actions, include a grocery shopping phase where you 'buy' ingredients for a meal for additional immersion. This practice mimics real-life scenarios where you might use ASL in addition to reinforcing the signs. It's a fantastic method to practice and gain confidence while utilizing these indicators in regular situations.

CHAPTER 9: SEASONS, WEATHER, AND NATURE-RELATED SIGNS

This chapter examines the colorful signs in American Sign Language (ASL) that relate to the environment, the weather, and the seasons. It's essential to recognize these cues in order to participate in regular discussions about our surroundings. You are advised to practice these signs in order to become proficient in communicating these basic components of nature in ASL. Each sign is explained in depth.

- **Spring**

Description: To sign 'spring,' it is sufficient to use the first part of the 'gardening' sign. Unlike the latter, however, the simulation of the plant emerging from the earth should be done repeatedly.

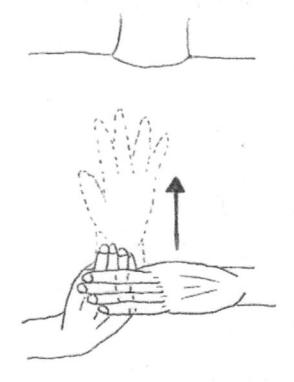

- **Summer**

Description: The ASL sign for "summer" is making a hand motion across your forehead that resembles wiping perspiration from your brow, changing from a "1" to a "x" form.

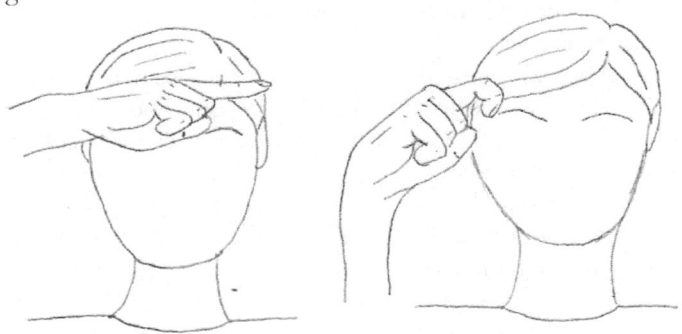

- **Autumn/Fall**

Description: Holding your non-dominant arm obliquely in front of your chest, slide your dominant hand along the lower part of the non-dominant forearm.

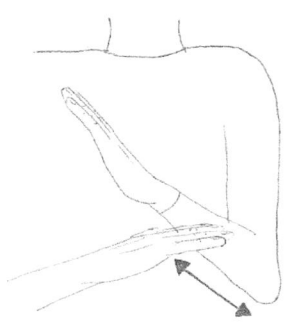

- **Winter**

Description: Similar to 'cold,' it is enough to shake your arms as if you are shivering, but in a more vigorous manner to differentiate it from 'cold.'

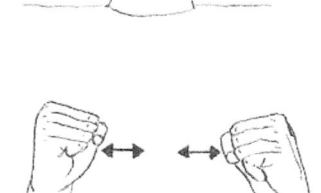

- **Rain**

Description: With the palms of your hands facing in front of you, lower both arms as if to simulate falling rain.

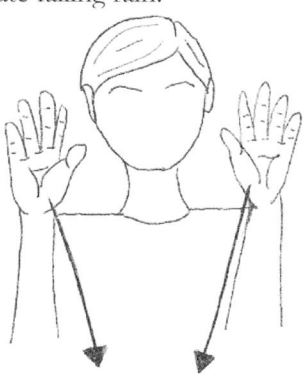

- **Snow**

Description: Very similar to 'rain,' but starting with your hands slightly lower, lower both arms downwards while moving all your fingers, as if to imitate falling snow.

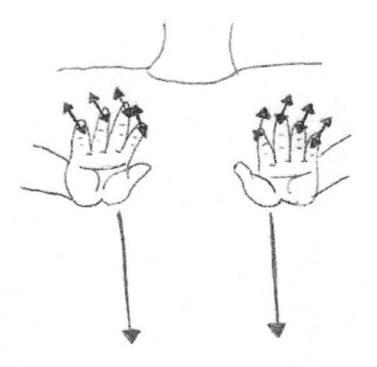

- **Wind**

Description: Holding your hands parallel to each other, gently shake them from right to left, imitating the blowing of the wind.

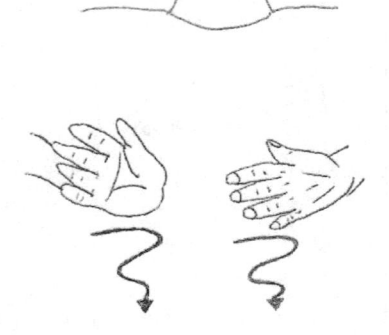

- **Sun**

Description: Flatten a "O" hand form and rotate it once in a circular motion. Then, open up the handshape by lowering it slightly.

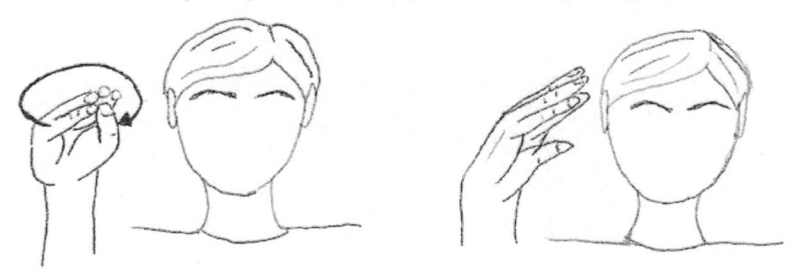

- **Tree**

Description: Extend your dominant arm upwards with the elbow bent and the hand flat, representing the trunk and branches of a tree. The dominant arm should rest on the back of the non-dominant hand.

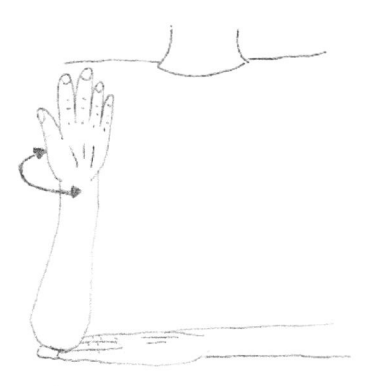

These signs offer a basic means of bringing up numerous topics related to weather, seasons, and the natural world in ASL. They boost your ability to understand and interpret events that occur in the natural world in addition to increasing your vocabulary.

Practical Exercise

Here's a practical exercise to help you better absorb these principles. Establish a specific amount of time each day for describing the weather and season in ASL. Use the indicators you've studied to describe the present season and weather, or just look out your window. For instance, use the signs for "winter" and "snow" to depict the outside view if it's a snowy winter day. Regular use of these signs will help you remember them better and improve your ability to use ASL in casual talks about the surroundings. As you gain confidence, try including more signs or descriptive parts to make longer, more complicated phrases.

BOOK 3: ADVANCED SKILLS IN ASL
CHAPTER 1: DESCRIBING PEOPLE: APPEARANCE AND PERSONALITY

The complex topic of characterizing people's appearance and personalities in American Sign Language (ASL) is the subject of this chapter. These indications point the way to more sophisticated communication abilities, which enable you to give thorough explanations and have deeper discussions. In ASL, precise and polite descriptions are essential to good interpersonal communication.

Tall/Short
- **Tall**

Description: Hold your non-dominant hand open with the palm facing outward. Slide your dominant hand with the index finger extended upward along the non-dominant hand.

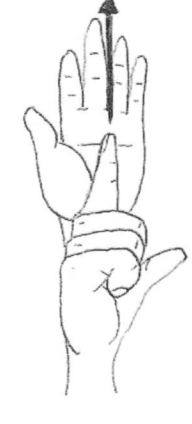

- **Short**

Description: Similarly to 'short,' place your hand flat and lower it downwards, but starting from a lower level than 'short'.

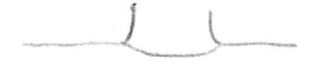

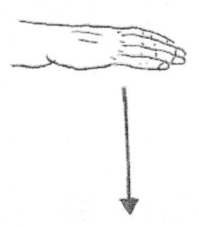

Hair (Length and Color)
- **Length**

Description: Put your palm where the hair ends to indicate the length of the hair (around the chin for short hair, lower for long hair).

- **Color**

Description: Point to your hair and use the fingerspelling technique to spell out the hair color.

- **Eye Color**

Description: Point to your eye and then use the fingerspelling technique to spell out the color.

- **Age**

Description: To indicate age, touch your chin with your hand closed in a fist and pull downwards, as if you were stretching a beard. Then, indicate the age by signing the corresponding number.

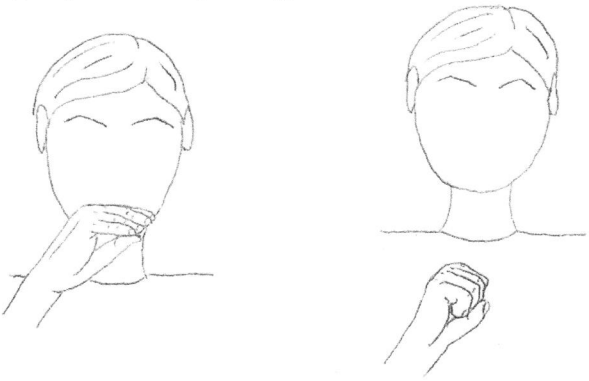

- **Serious**

Description: Place the indicated index below the lips, maintaining a facial expression, and move your hand slightly inward and outward.

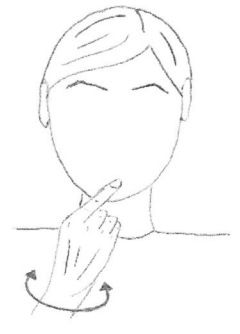

In ASL, describing someone is more than just describing their physical characteristics; it's about communicating a whole picture of the person. When utilized with consideration and respect, these indicators can promote a deeper level of understanding and connection in your relationships. Recall that the context in which you employ these signals and your facial expressions enhance the efficacy of your ASL communication.

Practical Exercise

Look at a family photo for a bit, or bring a close friend to mind. Try to give an ASL description of this individual using the signs you learned in this chapter. Begin with fundamental physical characteristics such as height, color, and length of hair, and proceed to eye color and age. Lastly, outline their character attributes. It's important to remember that your hand placement and facial expressions play a crucial role in communicating precise and courteous information in ASL. This exercise lets you practice integrating signs to make a thorough and courteous description of a person, in addition to testing your memory of individual signs.

CHAPTER 2: NAVIGATING: DIRECTIONS, PLACES, AND TRANSPORTATION

The navigation of different surroundings is the main subject of this chapter as we move into more advanced ASL topics. Knowing these signals will help you communicate more successfully in a variety of situations, from discussing transit options to asking for directions.

- **Left**

Description: Move your hand in a "L" shape to the left.

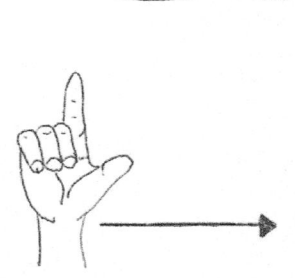

- **Right**

Description: In a similar manner, move your hand in a "R" shape to the right.

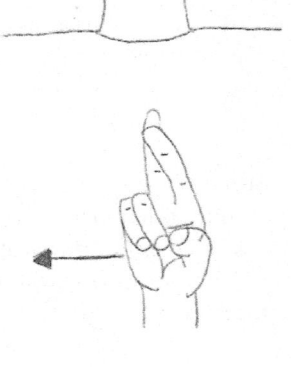

- **Straight**

Description: Lift one arm straight ahead and extend it in front of you.

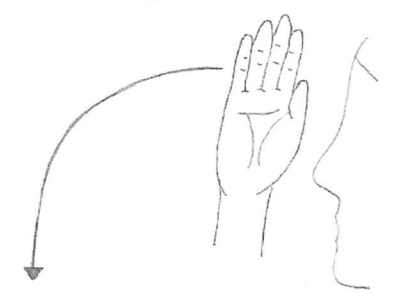

- **School**

Description: To make the sign "school," place your hands flat and quickly press your dominant hand down twice onto your base hand, creating the impression of clapping.

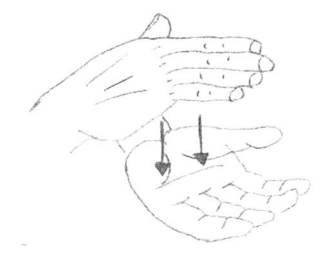

- **Train**

Description: In ASL, "train" is indicated by extending both hands' middle and index fingers. To simulate the action of a train traveling along railroad tracks, use the fingers of your dominant hand to slowly slide down the corresponding fingers of your non-dominant hand.

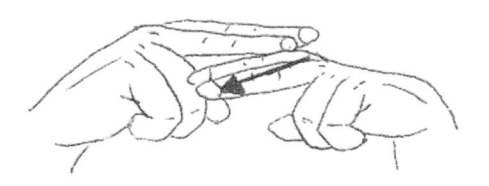

It takes more than just hand gestures to comprehend these ASL directions, location, and transit signs; you also need to be able to incorporate them into a smooth, educational dialogue. With these signals, you may have more in-depth conversations about navigating different situations, which enhances the depth and significance of your ASL interactions.

Interactive Scavenger Hunt Exercise

Make a straightforward scavenger hunt for your house or another familiar setting. Jot down a list of objects or places, such a window, a kitchen, or a book. Next, give yourself directions to each item or location using the ASL signs you have learnt in this chapter. Sign "straight" along the hallway, "left" at a hallway, and "right" into the kitchen, for instance. In addition to giving you practice, this activity pushes you to apply the signs in real-world situations, which will strengthen your understanding and help you become more fluent in everyday communication. Keep in mind that the secret to producing a dynamic and captivating ASL experience is to blend the signs together fluidly as you move about the room.

CHAPTER 3: PLANNING EVENTS AND ACTIVITIES

You can expand your proficiency in American Sign Language (ASL) by using it for event and activity planning and discussion. Signage pertaining to dates, hours, events, and event planning is covered in detail in this chapter. With the help of these signs, you can plan events, make appointments, and communicate about them clearly and precisely.

- **Event/Party**

Description: First, use both hands to make the letter "Y" in ASL. Touch your chest first, and then swiftly slide both hands lower and outward.

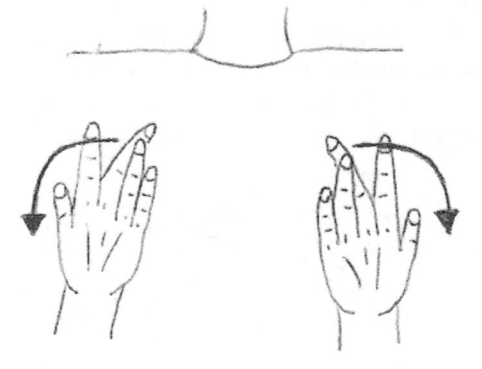

- **Date (Calendar Date)**

Description: Spell out the specific month using ASL fingerspelling, followed by the date using ASL number signs.

- **Time (Clock Time)**

Description: As though pointing to a watch, point to your wrist, and then indicate the time with numerical signs.

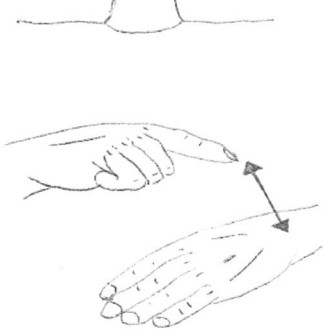

- **Schedule/Plan**

Description: With your hand open in a "4" shape, raise it in front of you to shoulder height. Then lower it from top to bottom and from inside to outside in a single, fluid motion.

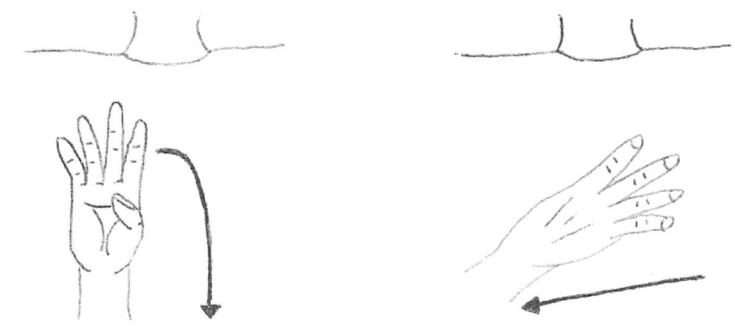

- **Meeting**

Description: Hold both hands at chest height, slightly open. Close and open your hands repeatedly while the fingers touch each other.

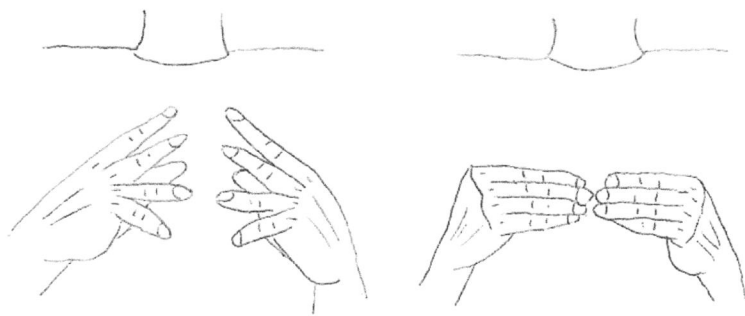

- **Vacation**

Description: To indicate "vacation," place your thumbs close to, but separated from, your armpits, and press them against your chest. When this sign is made once, it signifies "time off" or "off work," but when it is made twice, it implies a real "vacation" or "period of not working."

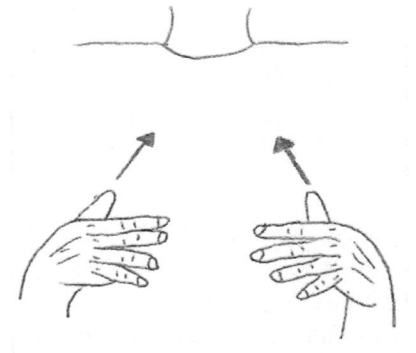

Learning these signs improves your social interactions as well as your ability to plan and discuss activities in ASL. With the use of these signs, you can more effectively and versatilely communicate in ASL by bridging the gap between basic conversational skills and more complicated language functions.

Practical Exercise

1. Create a mock event: Arrange a hypothetical occurrence using the indicators you learnt in this chapter. Using the "Event/Party" markers, provide a description of the event that includes the "Date" and "Time." Plan a birthday celebration, for instance, and use ASL to indicate the day, month, and hour.

2. Schedule a meeting: Enact a fictitious meeting to practice using the 'Schedule/Plan' indication. Indicate who will be present and when the meeting is scheduled by using the 'Meeting' indicator.

3. Plan a vacation: Write about your ideal vacation using the 'Vacation' sign. Using the relevant ASL signs, include information on the length of the vacation and your plans.

You can improve your recall and accuracy of these signs in real-world scenarios by actively applying them in a simulated context. This exercise enhances the subtlety and efficacy of your ASL communication by bridging the theory and practice gaps.

CHAPTER 4: AGREEING AND DISAGREEING IN ASL

Expressing agreement or disagreement is often a necessary part of effective communication. This is accomplished in American Sign Language (ASL) by using body language and facial emotions in addition to certain signs. The subtleties of agreeing and disagreeing in ASL are examined in this chapter, which is an essential component of advanced conversational abilities.

- **Agree/Yes**

Description: Start by closing both hands into fists, leaving only the index finger extended on each hand. The dominant hand's index finger should point to the head before moving to take its place next to the non-dominant hand that is being held in front of you.

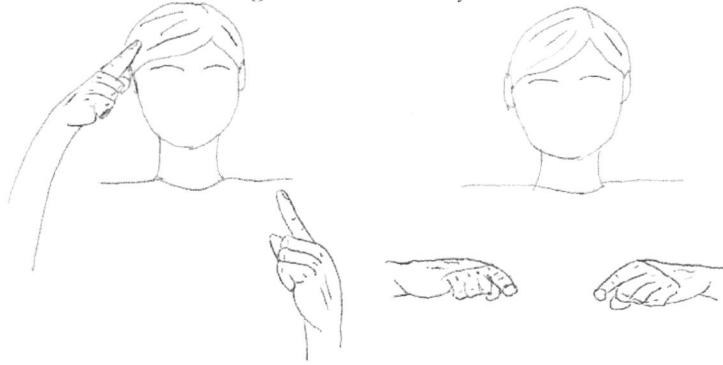

- **Disagree/No**

Description: The first part of the movement is identical to "agree." In the second part, however, after bringing the index fingers close in front of you, you need to make a movement with both hands outward.

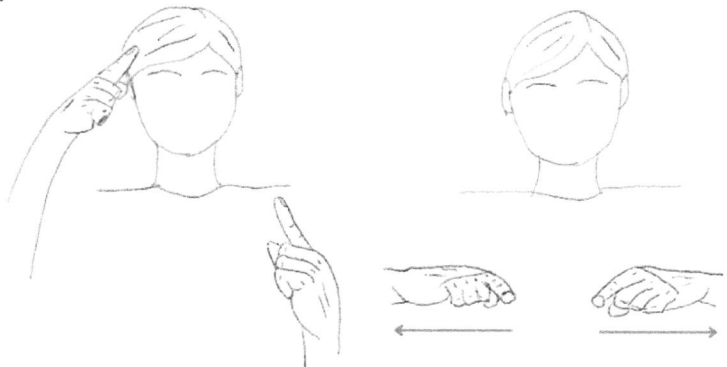

- **Understand/Comprehend**

Description: The movement is very similar to that of "don't understand" as seen in the previous chapters. The only difference is that the head remains still instead of shaking "no" as in "I don't understand."

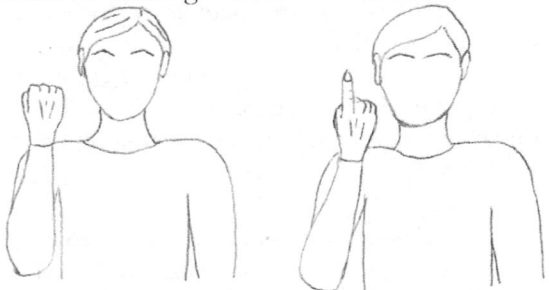

- **Confused**

Description: With your dominant hand, point to your forehead while the other hand remains open in front of you. Then bring your dominant hand close to the non-dominant one and rotate them together, maintaining a confused and bewildered facial expression.

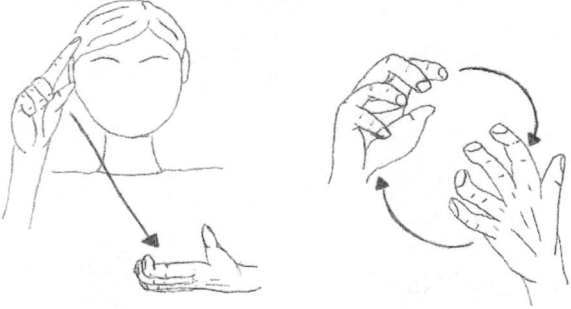

- **Exactly/Correct**

Description: Shape both of your hands into fists while extending only your index fingers. Place your dominant fist above the other one at an angle, and point towards the person you're conversing with as if to indicate, "You're correct!"

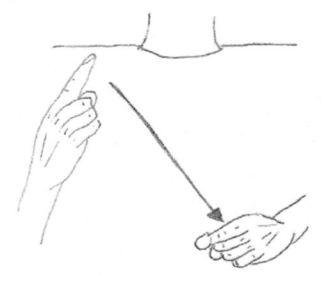

- **Wrong/Incorrect**

Description: Place the "Y"-shaped hand up against your chin.

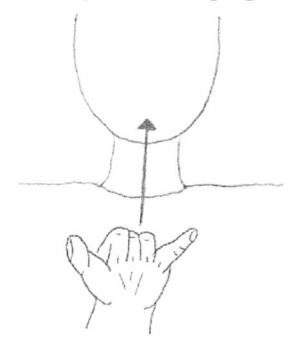

Being able to recognize and use these signals in ASL improves your ability to participate in sophisticated discussions, whether you're expressing agreement or disagreement or just wanting to be sure you understand something. Keep in mind that body language and facial emotions in ASL are just as crucial to communicating your message as the signs themselves.

Reflective Conversation Practice

Find a companion, someone who knows the language or another ASL learner. Have a straightforward discussion about themes that tend to elicit agreement or disagreement. During the discussion, use the appropriate signs to indicate your agreement or disagreement: "Agree/Yes," "Disagree/No," "Understand/Comprehend," "Confused," "Exactly/Correct," and "Wrong/Incorrect." Verify that the signs you are employing correspond with your facial expressions and body language. Take careful note of this. Pay close attention to this. Discuss with your buddy how well you were able to convey these ideas in ASL after the talk. Your capacity to express complex thoughts and understandings in ASL will improve as a result of this activity, which is essential for advanced conversational abilities.

CHAPTER 5: EXPRESSING LIKES, DISLIKES, AND PREFERENCES

In the complex world of American Sign Language (ASL), being able to communicate one's own preferences, aversions, and tastes is essential. In order to facilitate more expressive and customized interactions, this chapter explores the particular ASL signals and motions that are used to communicate preferences, dislikes, and likes.

- **Like**

Description: As already illustrated in Chapter 3 of Book Two, to indicate "like," start by signing "I" by pointing to yourself. Then touch your chest with an open hand, and as you move it away, sign the number "8."

- **Dislike**

Description: Start with your dominant hand facing towards you. Touch your chest with your thumb and middle finger together, then release your hand. As you move it away, rotate your wrist outward and fully open your hand, as if you are throwing something.

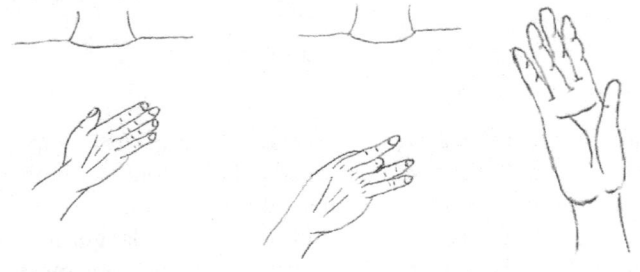

- **Prefer**

Description: Twice, the middle finger lightly taps the chin.

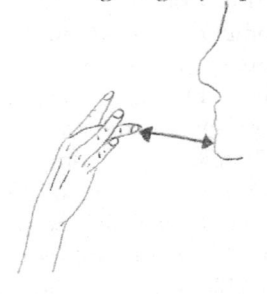

- **Interested**

Description: When you sign "interest" or "interested," start by making the "5" hand shape with both hands close to your chest and stomach, the dominant hand being higher. As you advance both hands, form the "8" shape with them.

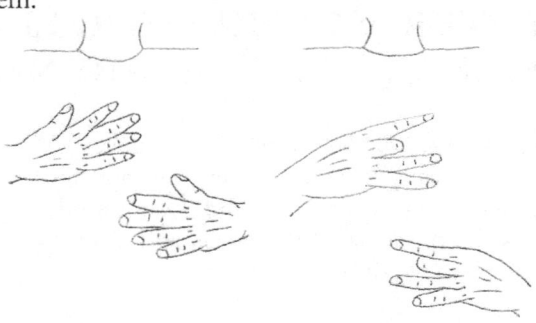

- **Bored**

Description: Your finger goes to the outside of your nose in this sign. Your finger should make a double twist gesture to indicate "boring."

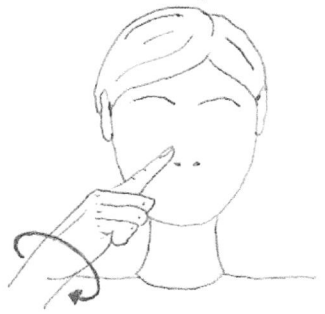

Building relationships and exchanging personal insights require the ability to communicate preferences, dislikes, and likes in American Sign Language (ASL). These indicators deepen discussions and promote a more lively flow of thoughts and feelings.

Practical Exercise

Use ASL to create a little video journal entry or diary. Share your thoughts, opinions, and likes and dislikes on a range of subjects in this video. You might talk about your favorite meals, movies, pastimes, or everyday routines. As you talk about each topic, use the signals for "like," "dislike," "prefer," "interested," and "bored." To effectively communicate emotions and preferences in ASL, pay close attention to how you complement your signs with your body language and facial expressions. Watch your video when it's finished to evaluate how well you used signs and how clear your expression was. This practice helps you express your own preferences and emotions in ASL more effectively while also reinforcing the signs.

CHAPTER 6: INTERROGATIVE WORDS AND FORMULATING QUESTIONS IN ASL

One of the more challenging aspects of learning American Sign Language (ASL) is navigating the structure and nuances of question formulation. An essential component of efficient ASL communication, question construction is covered in great detail in this chapter. Basic interrogative signals such as 'who,' 'where,' 'what,' 'when,' 'why,' and 'how' have already been covered in Chapter 1, "ESSENTIAL SIGNS FOR DAILY COMMUNICATION" in Book 2, so we won't go over them again here. Rather, we turn our attention to the skill of building questions in ASL, fusing these interrogative signs with other linguistic components to produce queries that are understandable, logical, and appropriate for the given situation.

As a visual language, ASL mostly uses body language, facial expressions, and sign order to transmit meaning. In contrast to English, where a sentence's structure frequently establishes whether it is a statement or a question, ASL does this through the use of non-manual indicators such head tilts and eyebrow motions. Anybody hoping to communicate well in ASL must be aware of these nuances.

The eyebrows hold the key when it comes to yes/no questions. Often, a yes/no question is indicated by raised eyebrows and an inquiring gaze. These types of inquiries typically have the verb appear before the topic in ASL.

- **Example 1**: "GO you STORE?" (accompanied by raised eyebrows) translates to "Are you going to the store?" in English. Here, the verb 'GO' precedes the subject 'you.'

Wh- questions (who, what, where, when, why, and how) in ASL involve incorporating the specific 'Wh-' sign at either the beginning or the end of the sentence. Unlike yes/no questions, these questions typically use furrowed brows.

- **Example 2**: "WHERE LIBRARY?" with furrowed brows asks, "Where is the library?" You can put the "WHERE" indicator at the beginning or conclusion of the statement.
- **Example 3**: "YOU NAME WHAT?" Here, the question word 'WHAT' comes at the end, asking "What is your name?"

In ASL, answering questions usually entails repeating the verb that was posed. For example, a simple "GO" and a nod can be enough to indicate yes when asked, "GO you STORE?"

Multiple elements may be combined in more complicated ASL questions. Take the question, "YOUR BIRTHDAY WHEN?" (Your birthday is when?) blends the declarative (YOUR BIRTHDAY) with the interrogative (WHEN).

In ASL, context is extremely important. The conversational context can influence the meaning of identical signs. This is particularly true with questions, as the context, the speakers' relationship, and the surrounding discourse all affect how the signs are interpreted.

Learning the complex web of facial expressions, body language, and contextual signals that make up ASL's visual language is equally as important as mastering the signs. All these factors interact when asking questions in ASL effectively, facilitating a more in-depth and complex exchange of ideas.

For those who want to improve their ASL questioning abilities, this chapter offers a strong starting point. Practice is the key to acquiring any language. Asking and understanding questions in ASL will become much easier with the help of native ASL speakers, ASL content, and consistent practice. All of these activities will enhance your general communication skills in ASL.

Recall that learning ASL fluency is a marathon, not a sprint. Acquiring expertise in features such as question creation is a first step toward developing a closer connection with the lively Deaf community and its rich cultural tapestry, in addition to linguistic proficiency.

CHAPTER 7: UNDERSTANDING AND USING NON-MANUAL MARKERS FOR CLARITY

American Sign Language (ASL) incorporates a variety of non-manual markers (NMMs) that are essential to communication in addition to the manual dexterity of hands creating signs. Body language, eye contact, head movements, and facial emotions are examples of NMMs. Each of these cues gives the signs additional emotional depth and context. By breaking down these essential elements, this chapter will help you communicate more effectively in ASL than just with hand gestures.

- **Facial Expressions**

In ASL, facial emotions are essential components of meaning communication, not just decorative elements. They can convey the meaning, tone, and intent of a sign.

Examples and Contexts

1. Eyebrow Position: Raised eyebrows often indicate a yes/no question, while furrowed brows are used for WH-questions (who, what, where, when, why, how).

2. Mouth Shapes: In ASL, mouth gestures can be used to indicate adjectives or adverbs. A closed mouth, for instance, may convey a little size or distance, whereas an open mouth may convey a huge size or intensity.

3. Eye Gaze: Making eye contact is essential to ASL. Maintaining eye contact demonstrates respect and engagement, whereas breaking it might convey discomfort or disinterest.

- **Head Movements**

Head movements give the signs more clarity and intensity. They have the option to confirm, deny, or contest the information being signed.

Examples and Contexts

1. Nodding: A nod while signing can emphasize agreement or affirmation.

2. Shaking Head: A head shake while signing indicates negation or disagreement.

3. Tilting Head: A tilt can indicate curiosity, confusion, or be used for emphasis.

- **Body Posture and Movement**

The orientation and movement of your body can provide context and indicate subjects and objects within a conversation.

Examples and Contexts

1. Leaning Forward: This can show interest or emphasis in the conversation.

2. Shifting Body: Shifting from side to side can indicate different subjects or aspects of a conversation.

3. Upper Body: The movement of the upper body can mimic the action being described, adding a visual element to the description.

- **Eye Gaze**

You may determine the subject, object, or direction of action in a statement in ASL by looking in a certain direction. It's a subdued yet effective method for increasing clarity.

Examples and Contexts

1. Looking at the Hand: Indicates focusing on the action or subject being signed about.

2. Looking Away: Can be used to indicate reflection, recalling information, or sometimes disengagement.

3. Directional Gaze: Gazing in a particular direction while signing can indicate the location or direction of the subject matter.

- **Incorporating NMMs in Conversation**

Using NMMs in your ASL talks enhances the communication and gives it a more genuine and expressive quality. When you pose a question, for example, your expression should be appropriate for the question. In a similar vein, your facial expression should convey the emotion you are portraying.

It's just as vital to learn ASL NMMs as it is to master the signs themselves. These markers give your interactions more depth and passion by expressing subtleties that signs alone are unable to communicate. You can improve the dynamic, expressive, and nuanced nature of your ASL communication by comprehending and skillfully applying NMMs.

Keep an eye out for these non-manual signals as you continue to study and practice ASL. You can get much better at signing by watching native signers, practicing in front of a mirror, and using NMMs in your regular signing. Keep in mind that ASL is an expressive and visual language, and these non-manual components are essential to making your interactions engaging.

BOOK 4: PRACTICAL AND FUNCTIONAL ASL
CHAPTER 1: SIGNS FOR EMERGENCY SITUATIONS AND HEALTH

Knowing how to properly communicate in an emergency and address health-related matters in the context of American Sign Language (ASL) is not only advantageous—it may even save lives. As a crucial component of the "Practical and Functional ASL" portion, this chapter focuses on providing students with the necessary signs for health and emergency situations. In urgent circumstances, knowing these indicators and knowing when to apply them can have significant implications.

- **Emergency**

Description: Shape your dominant hand into the ASL letter E sign and wriggle it from side to side.

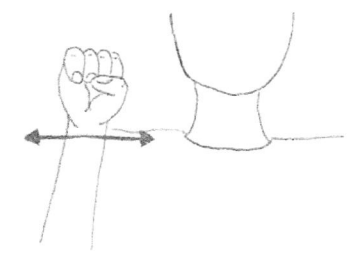

- **Pain**

Description: Bring your hands close to each other with only the index fingers extended. In this position, rotate the dominant hand downward and the non-dominant hand upward, as if the two index fingers are screwing in opposite directions from each other.

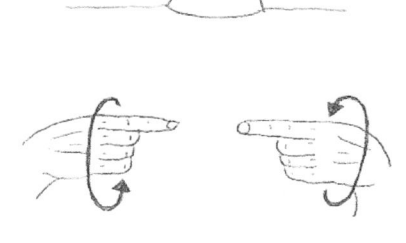

- **Doctor**

Description: Slide the fingers of your dominant hand across the palm of your non-dominant hand.

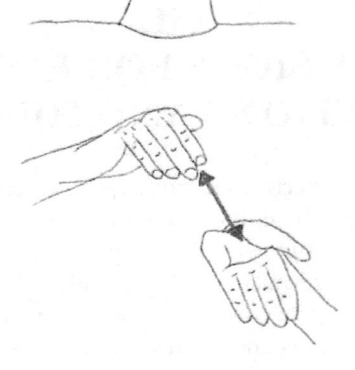

- **Hospital**

Description: Make a "cross" shape with the "H" handshape on your shoulder.

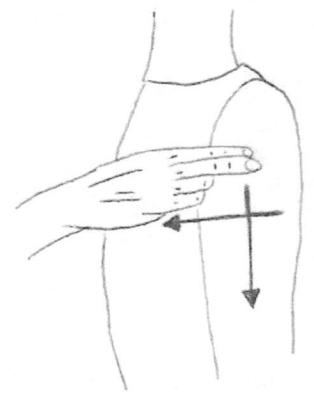

- **Medicine/Medication**

Description: After placing your right hand's middle finger on your left hand's palm, turn your right hand to the other side several times.

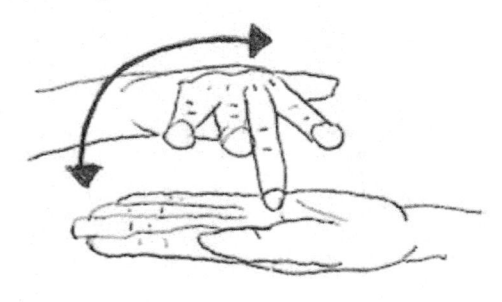

- **Allergy**

Description: With your dominant hand's index finger, start by touching your nose. Then bring both thumbs close together in an oblique position and move them away from each other.

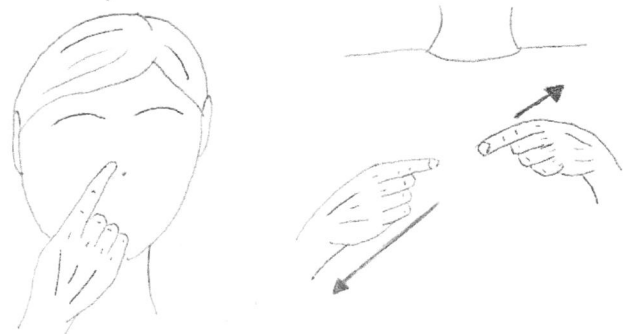

- **Accident**

Description: Start with both hands open and the palms facing you. Conclude by bringing the two fists together in front of your chest.

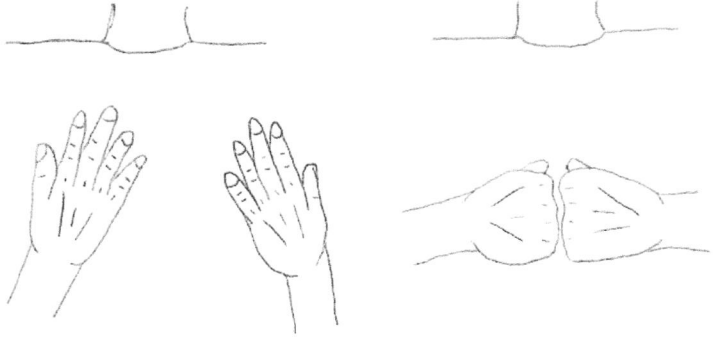

Being proficient in these signs can significantly improve your capacity to communicate during crises and severe health circumstances. Clear and timely communication is crucial in these situations, and ASL can frequently fill in the gaps where spoken words can fall short. These signs serve a purpose beyond simple information delivery: they guarantee people's health, safety, and well-being when they need it most.

Knowing when to use each of these signals and practicing them on a regular basis can help you be ready for situations where prompt and clear communication is needed. It's crucial to keep in mind that nonverbal clues and expressions are crucial in communicating the seriousness and urgency of an emergency. Adding these signs to your repertoire as you continue to learn ASL can help you become not just a skilled signer but also an invaluable communicator during emergencies.

Practical Exercise: Role-Playing for Emergency Scenarios

Take part in a role-playing activity to solidify your comprehension of and proficiency with these signs. You can practice alone or in pairs with another learner in front of a mirror. Act out different emergency situations. For example, play out what it might be like to be in pain, need medical attention, or have an accident. In these situations, use the proper signals for "help," "emergency," "pain," "doctor," "hospital," "medicine/medication," "allergy," and "accident." Make sure your body language and facial emotions reflect the gravity and urgency of each circumstance. Through this activity, you will not only learn the signs and how to apply them while communicating clearly and quickly in real-life situations, but you will also improve your memory of them. Keep in mind that being able to communicate clearly and swiftly might be crucial in emergency situations.

CHAPTER 2: SIGN LANGUAGE IN EDUCATION AND THE WORKPLACE

In today's changing world American Sign Language (ASL) is essential in both educational and professional contexts. This chapter focuses on ASL signs that are very helpful in professional and academic settings. Comprehending and applying these indicators can effectively close gaps in communication, promote inclusion, and improve teamwork in heterogeneous environments.

- **Learn**

Description: Put your non-dominant hand's palm in front of you. Next, use your dominant hand to lightly touch your forehead, as though you were taking something and putting it in the palm of your non-dominant hand.

- **Teach**

Description: This symbol starts close to your head and spreads outward, seemingly representing the idea of sending information from your mind to another person's.

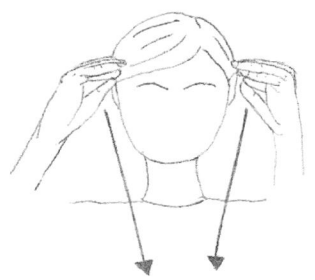

- **Class**

Description: Make a 'C' form with your hands and move them together in a circular motion, as you are encircling a class or group.

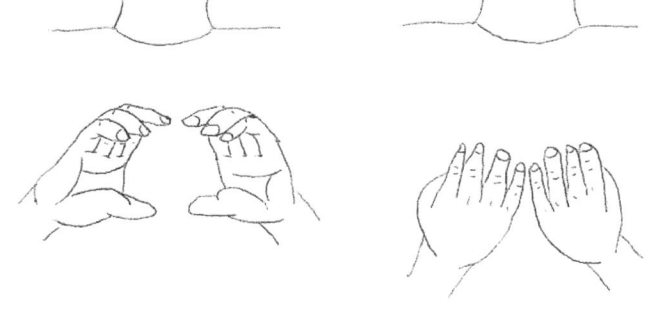

- **Project**

Description: Open your non-dominant hand with the palm facing you. Start by signing "2" with your dominant hand, and from behind the non-dominant hand, make a movement as if to leap over it. Once leaped over, change the position of your dominant hand by keeping only the little finger extended and sliding it along the back of your non-dominant hand.

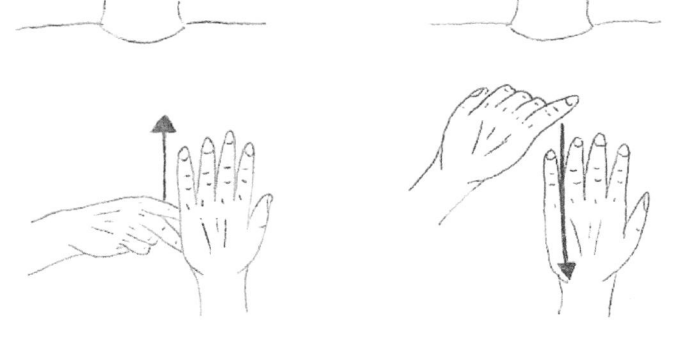

- **Deadline**

Description: Make a hand gesture that represents severing your throat to indicate a deadline or cutoff time.

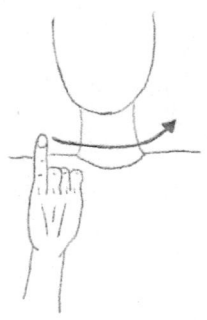

Understanding these indicators can greatly improve communication in academic and professional settings, leading to more inclusive and productive interactions. In these contexts, ASL is about more than simply individual communication; it's about fostering an atmosphere where everyone, deaf or not, has equal access to resources and chances for participation.

Exercise: Create a Short ASL Presentation

Create a concise ASL presentation that includes the following signs: "Learn," "Teach," "Class," "Project," "Team/Group," and "Deadline." This might be regarding a team project, a class you're taking, or an ongoing endeavor. Make use of each indicator to explain a different facet of your subject. For instance, give an explanation of a recent learning, impart a crucial idea, characterize the dynamics of the group, delineate the parameters of the project, and bring up any significant due dates. Try recording yourself so you can review and improve your sign language skills. This practice will assist with learning these particular signs by heart as well as with comprehending how to utilize ASL in practical situations.

CHAPTER 3: SIGNS FOR SHOPPING, MONEY, AND TRANSACTIONS

Purchasing things and making money transactions are essential aspects of daily living. In these circumstances, it is imperative that users of American Sign Language (ASL) communicate intelligibly. Comprehensive instructions on ASL signs for money, shopping, and other transactions are given in this chapter. Being proficient with these indicators improves one's capacity to move independently and with confidence through operations.

- **Sell**

Description: Put your fingers and thumb together in front of you, then extend your wrists forward.

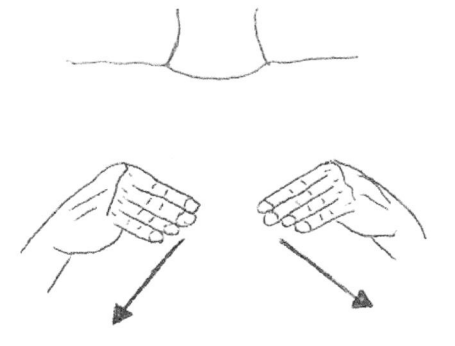

- **Money**

Description: To sign "money," take your hand and make a flattened "O" shape, like you're holding some cash. Tape it lightly twice on the palm of your other hand.

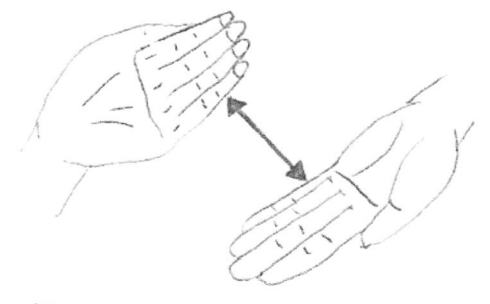

- **Price/Cost**

Description: To sign "price," hold your non-dominant hand out straight in front of you plain. With your dominant hand forming a "X" with the palm facing back, strike the palm of your non-dominant hand with the tip of your "X" finger by moving downward.

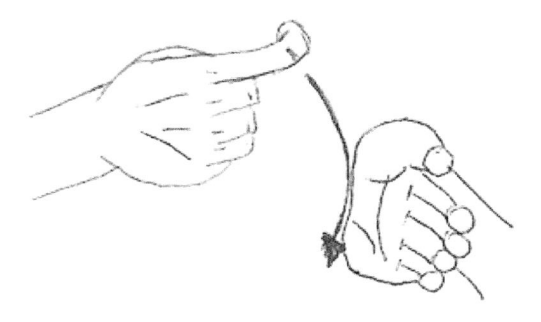

- **Expensive**

Description: Transfer a flattened "O" hand to your left palm, lift it, and bring it down in a throwing motion while opening it fast into a loose form.

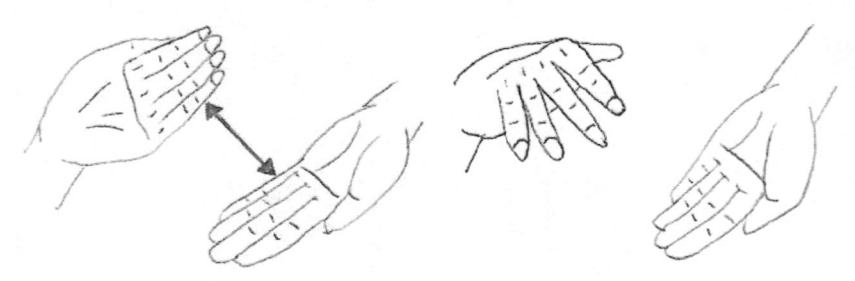

- **Cheap**

Description: With one hand raised vertically in front of you, gently brush the palm of the vertical hand with the other as you slide it from top to bottom.

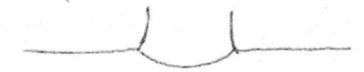

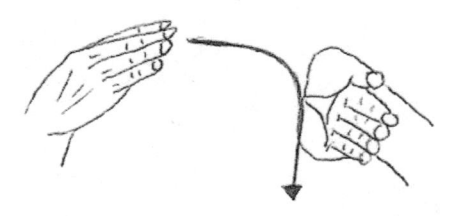

- **Credit Card**

Description: With your non-dominant hand open and facing up, slide the fist across the open palm.

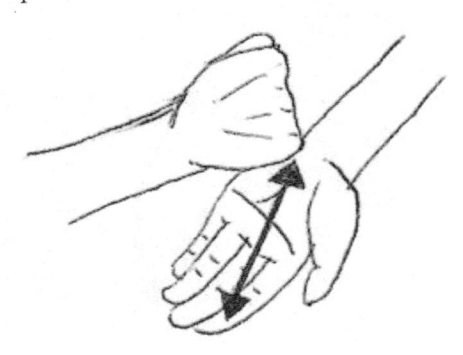

- **Receipt**

Description: Imitate a receipt by sliding both of your hands vertically in the shape of a slip.

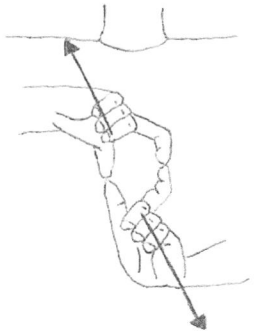

Knowing these indicators makes it easier to conduct financial and shopping transactions, and it also gives people the confidence to fully engage in these daily activities. Being able to sign a variety of shopping and money-related issues is essential for efficient and clear ASL communication.

Practical Exercise: ASL Shopping Scenario Simulation

At home, set up a fictitious shopping scenario. Get a few things to stand in for various products, and you can use real or play money. Try out each of the following signs: "Sell," "Money," "Price/Cost," "Expensive," "Cheap," "Credit Card," and "Receipt." This is a simulated shopping experience. To question the price of an object, for example, pick it up, use the 'Price/Cost' sign, and then answer with the appropriate sign, such as 'Expensive' or 'Cheap.' After feigning to pay with "Money" or a "Credit Card," sign the "Receipt."

By placing the signs in their natural environment, this activity improves your memory and practical use of the signs in real-world shopping and transaction scenarios.

CHAPTER 4: PROVIDING INSTRUCTIONS AND DIRECTIONS

Effectively conveying instructions and directions is a fundamental ability in American Sign Language (ASL). This chapter explores indicators that are essential for conveying instructions, explaining processes, and directing others in a variety of situations. These ASL signals will improve your ability to convey instructions effectively, whether you're leading someone to a place, outlining a task, or assisting them through a procedure.

- **Go/Move**

Description: Point your index fingers forward and move your hands in the direction you're indicating.

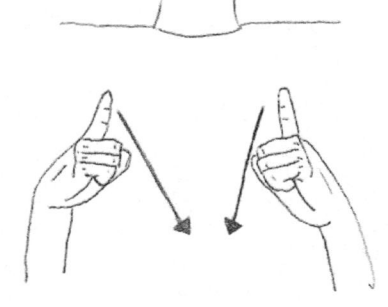

- **Stop/Halt**

Description: When you sign "stop," extend your left hand palm up and quickly bring your open right hand down to meet the left palm, creating a right angle.

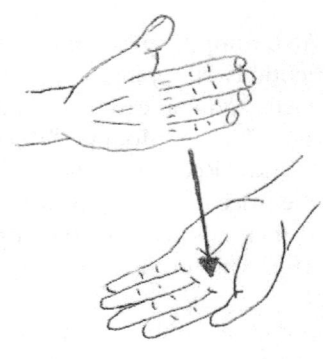

- **Turn**

Description: Hold your dominant hand in an "L" shape and rotate it in the direction you want to indicate the turn.

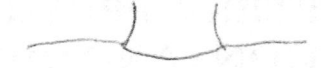

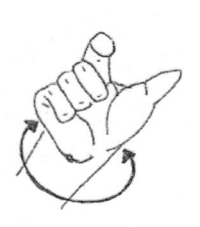

- **Here**

Description: With the fingers pointed down and the palms facing outward, open your hands. While maintaining this position, rotate both hands in a synchronized motion.

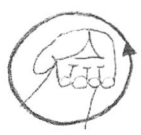

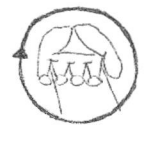

- **There**

Description: Position your dominant hand with the palm facing upward, as if you are carrying a tray. While maintaining this position, move your arm forward.

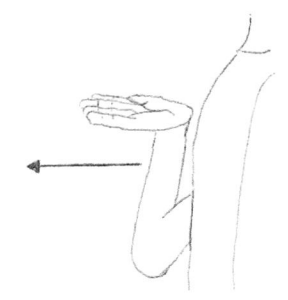

- **Up/Down**

Description: Point and move your index finger upward to indicate "up." Point and move it down to indicate "down."

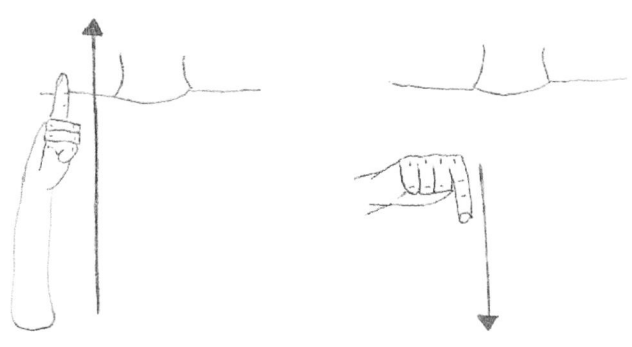

- **Follow**

Description: Keeping your thumbs raised, close your fists and push them outward from your chest.

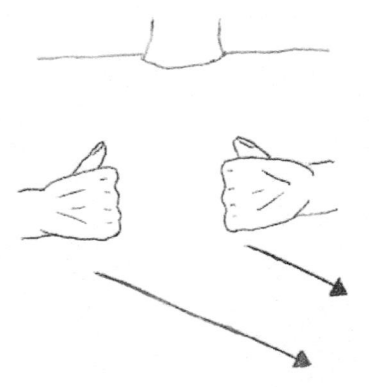

- **Show/Explain**

Description: Using the index finger of your dominant-hand, open the other hand vertically and touch its palm. Holding this position, both hands go forward.

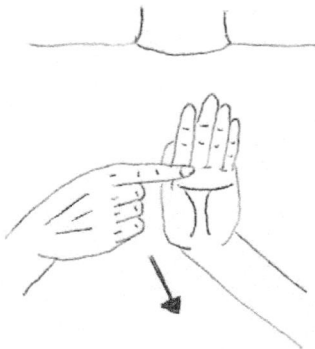

It is important to ensure clarity and comprehension in communication by comprehending and utilizing these signs to provide instructions and suggestions in ASL. These indicators are particularly helpful in a variety of contexts, from social situations to more technical settings like offices or classrooms.

Exercise: Create a Directional Story in ASL

Using the signs you learnt in this chapter, create a short tale. The narrative should center on a character being led by multiple sets of instructions and directives from one place to another. Using signs for "go," "turn," "stop," and other commands, for example, describe a person traveling from their house to a neighboring café. Practice signing this narrative, paying attention to your gestures' flow and clarity. This practice helps you become more proficient at communicating in ASL by reinforcing the signs and strengthening your ability to put them together in a meaningful story. Recall that the objective is to use the signals you've learned to tell the story succinctly and clearly.

CHAPTER 5: PRACTICE STRATEGIES AND LEARNING RESOURCES

Learning American Sign Language (ASL) is a rewarding endeavor that provides a plethora of new opportunities for communication. This long chapter, tucked away in the "Practical and Functional ASL" section, is devoted to providing a wealth of practice techniques and a variety of learning materials. Being proficient in ASL requires more than just learning signs; it also entails comprehending the subtleties of a language that is intricately linked to the experiences and culture of the Deaf community. We'll get into specific techniques and tools that help promote a deeper comprehension and competency in ASL here.

In-Depth Practice Strategies
1. **Daily Sign Usage**: One of the best strategies to improve fluency is to incorporate ASL into your everyday activities. Start by substituting signs for frequently used verbal phrases. Practice your signals for things like "good morning," "breakfast," and "today" when you first wake up. As you advance, set a goal for yourself to have full ASL discussions, even in front of a mirror or with yourself. This continuous interaction aids in helping your memory retain signs and their meanings.
2. **Mirroring and Feedback**: You can view your signals as others would by practicing in front of a mirror, which will change the way you perceive the forms and motions of your hands. Watching and recording videos can help you catch errors and subtleties that you would miss in live practice. Ask knowledgeable ASL users or teachers for their opinions. Giving yourself constructive criticism might help you improve your signature and steer clear of frequent mistakes.
3. **Role-playing Scenarios**: Make up scenarios based on things you would come across in real life or in particular places, such as a restaurant, doctor's office, or workplace. If at all possible, run through these scenarios with a partner. This approach increases your comfort in using ASL in a variety of contexts and helps you get ready for discussions in the real world. Since you may be imaginative with the events you play out, it's also a fun method to learn.

Learning Resources
1. **Deaf Community Events**: Getting involved with the Deaf community is incredibly beneficial. Attend workshops, events, and get-togethers for the Deaf community in your area. Speaking with ASL native speakers will provide you a real-world introduction to the language. In order to comprehend the context and etiquette of ASL, it also offers insight into the Deaf culture. These gatherings are frequently friendly and offer excellent chances to hone your abilities in a safe setting.
2. **ASL Clubs and Practice Groups**: Whether they meet in person or virtually, joining an ASL club or group can greatly accelerate your learning. These programs provide an organized method of practicing ASL and are frequently run by seasoned signers. They can offer a helpful setting for honing conversational skills, getting feedback, and exchanging pointers for learning.
3. **Volunteer Opportunities**: Look for volunteer positions at community centers, Deaf schools, or other establishments that assist the Deaf and hard of hearing where you can utilize ASL. This gives you real-world experience and lets you make a good impact on the community. One fulfilling method to advance your ASL proficiency and make a difference is by volunteering.

It takes constant practice and immersion to become proficient in ASL. You will improve your language abilities and obtain a deeper grasp of the rich culture and history of the Deaf community by using these specific tactics and interacting with the resources that are accessible within the Deaf community. Recall that the objective is to embrace and comprehend a dynamic culture and its distinct communication style, not just to acquire a language.

Learning ASL is an adventure that involves more than just communicating; it's about forming connections and fostering a diverse and active community. You get increasingly intimately acquainted with this exquisite language and the vibrant culture it symbolizes with each ASL discussion you have, every event you attend, and every encounter you have with the Deaf community. Remain devoted, maintain your curiosity, and savor each moment of this fulfilling trip.

CHAPTER 6: INTERACTING WITH THE DEAF COMMUNITY

Learning American Sign Language (ASL) and interacting with the Deaf community is a journey that breaks down language barriers and leads to a rich cultural experience. Understanding the intricacies and nuances of communicating with the Deaf community is essential to learning ASL, and it is the subject of this chapter. Here, the focus is on the manners, cultural norms, and successful communication techniques that are necessary for courteous and meaningful encounters rather than the signs themselves.

Deaf community is defined by its own set of cultural norms, values, and social customs. Acquiring knowledge of these facets is equally crucial as mastering ASL. Beyond just communicating, interacting with the Deaf community involves fostering relationships, appreciating other viewpoints, and enjoying a rich cultural legacy.

The Deaf community has a strong sense of identity, customs, the arts, and history, and they place a high importance on their language and culture. Members frequently use a capital "D" to denote their cultural identity in order to set it apart from the hearing impairment known as deafness.

Maintaining eye contact is important for proper communication etiquette in ASL because it shows respect and attentiveness. Essential elements of ASL are facial expressions and body language, which lend additional meaning and emotion to the signals. It's fine to give a Deaf person a gentle tap on the shoulder or a wave in their peripheral vision to grab their attention. It's important to be clear and patient while making sure your signs are clearly visible.

Being sensitive to cultural differences is essential when working with Deaf people. It is important to approach these contacts with an open mind, prepared to pick up on and comprehend the subtle cultural differences. Be receptive to learning about Deaf people's cultures and refrain from assuming anything about their abilities or preferences. It's also critical to acknowledge the variety within the Deaf community because Deaf people have a range of experiences and backgrounds.

Attending Deaf events provides an intensive setting for ASL practice and a deeper understanding of the Deaf community. It is best to observe first and then take an active part. Starting a conversation by introducing yourself and your ASL learning path can be very beneficial. Having conversations with ASL signers who are native speakers gives you a wealth of knowledge about the subtleties of the language. You may watch and pick up on the expressions that are used, the way the language flows naturally, and the cultural allusions.

Volunteering for groups that support the Deaf community can be a beneficial and gratifying method to practice ASL. It offers a place for interacting with other community members, getting to know their stories, and picking up tips from them. Respecting people's preferences for communication in every interaction—whether they prefer lipreading, signing, or utilizing an interpreter—is crucial. It demonstrates your regard for their culture and identity to acknowledge and respect their preferences.

Being in the company of the Deaf community is an amazing experience that goes beyond picking up a new language. It's about developing deep connections, accepting a fresh cultural viewpoint, and comprehending various experiences. There are many opportunities to deepen your awareness and admiration of this lively community as you embark on a journey of continual learning and growth into the Deaf community.

As you go with your ASL study and interactions with the Deaf community, keep in mind the significance of openness, respect, and cultural sensitivity. Every conversation is an opportunity to improve one's awareness of culture as well as one's linguistic abilities. If you approach this journey with an open mind and heart, you will discover that it is a deeply fulfilling experience.

CHAPTER 7: OVERCOMING COMMON CHALLENGES AND FRUSTRATIONS

Like learning any new language, learning American Sign Language (ASL) is an adventure with its own set of difficulties and frustrating moments. Learning ASL requires more than just memorizing grammar and signs; it also requires acclimating oneself to a new way of life and culture. This chapter promises to make learning easier and more pleasurable for newcomers by guiding them through common obstacles they may face and offering solutions.

Making the transition from a spoken to a visual language is one of the initial difficulties that many ASL learners encounter. ASL uses body language, gestures, and facial expressions to convey meaning instead of spoken languages, which use sounds. At first, this shift may be too much to handle since it calls for learning new signs as well as developing your ability to convey and read nonverbal messages. It is imperative to practice frequently and immerse oneself in the language as much as possible in order to overcome this. You can greatly enhance your comprehension and use of these non-verbal cues by practicing signing in front of a mirror, going to Deaf events, and watching films of native signers.

The quickness and fluidity of native signers is another frequent obstacle. The speed at which seasoned signers communicate might be intimidating to novices. It's crucial to keep in mind that ASL fluency requires time and practice, just like any other language. Learn the fundamentals of signs and phrases first, then progressively expand your vocabulary and comprehension. Never be afraid to request that signers repeat or slow down their signs. Above all, understand that becoming proficient is a slow process and practice self-patience.

Another area where novices frequently fail is finger spelling. It calls for accuracy and speed in word spelling as well as dexterity. Practice frequently, spell words you find around you, and take part in finger spelling exercises or games to get better at spelling with your fingers. Your accuracy and speed will increase with time, making it simpler to comprehend and interact in ASL.

Comprehension of ASL grammar can also be difficult. ASL's syntax and grammatical structure can diverge significantly from English's. For example, a topic-comment sentence structure in ASL may be foreign to beginning learners. Furthermore, practice with native signers might help you better understand how the language flows naturally.

A common source of dissatisfaction among novice learners is the apprehension of making errors. It's important not to forget that making inaccuracies is an inevitable component of learning. Every mistake is a teaching opportunity. In spite of your doubts about your signature, go ahead and sign. The Deaf community will value your efforts to learn their language and is normally highly supportive of people who are studying ASL.

Finally, ASL learners may find it difficult to understand cultural quirks. There are customs, traditions, and etiquette unique to the Deaf community. It is essential to comprehend these cultural nuances in order to communicate effectively. Spend some time learning about Deaf culture through literature, the internet, or conversations with other Deaf people. Your conversations with Deaf people will be more meaningful and your ASL abilities will improve as a result of this cultural awareness.

In conclusion, even though learning ASL can be difficult at times, it is completely feasible to get past these obstacles with perseverance, practice, and a desire to fully immerse oneself in the language and culture. Every accomplishment is a milestone, and every stride forward signifies progress. Accept the process of learning, and you'll quickly discover that your ASL communication is becoming more assured and efficient.

BOOK 5: INSIGHTS AND ADVANCED TOPICS IN ASL
CHAPTER 1: INTRODUCTION TO ASL GRAMMAR AND SYNTAX

Acquiring knowledge of American Sign Language (ASL) entails knowing not just the signs themselves but also the specific syntax and grammar that underpin them. This chapter explores the intricacies of syntax and grammar in ASL, which is crucial knowledge for anyone hoping to become fluent. Although ASL's basic sentence structure and non-manual markers were covered in earlier chapters, this section will go into further detail about other facets of the language, providing insights and more complex ideas.

ASL Sentence Structure

As was covered in previous chapters, the usual sentence form in ASL is "TOPIC" + "COMMENT". This structure reflects the visual-spatial aspect of the language and is very different from that of English. We won't go over the fundamentals again here, but it's crucial to keep in mind that ASL's structure prioritizes ideas above specifics when expressing concepts, as seen by the way concepts are presented.

Role Shifting

One vital and dynamic feature of ASL grammar is role shifting. It entails altering your facial expressions and body language to portray several characters or points of view within a story. This method is very important for narrating stories or transferring interpersonal conversations.

A signer must physically and expressively portray different personalities in order to use role shifting effectively. If you were narrating a story about a conversation between two persons, for example, you would move your body to one side to sign the dialogue of one person and to the other side to indicate the dialogue of the other. This gives the story more depth and clarity while also making it clearer who is speaking.

Role shifting is something that takes experience and attention to detail to understand and master. It all comes down to being able to switch between points of view with ease and convey each character's point of view effectively. This feature of ASL language creates a wealth of opportunities for compelling and expressive storytelling.

Facial Grammar

Facial expressions in ASL are more than merely emotional states, as was covered in previous chapters; they constitute a fundamental part of the language's grammatical structure. A sign's meaning can become more nuanced and sophisticated with each shift in facial expression. A raised eyebrow, for example, might be used to ask a question, while a furrowed brow can indicate focus or confusion.

Gaining a complete knowledge of facial grammar requires an understanding of how slight changes in facial expressions can change the meaning of a sign or remark. Both ASL expression and comprehension depend on this information. Students should practice both the signals and the appropriate facial expressions in order to convey their message clearly.

Fingerspelling

Although fingerspelling has already discussed, it is still worth examining. It is employed to spell names, locations, or particular terms that lack an ASL sign. It serves as a bridge between ASL and English, enabling the clear delivery of certain information.

Learners should practice fingerspelling swiftly and smoothly, making sure that each letter is clear, to develop their skills. Knowing when to utilize fingerspelling in ASL talks is also crucial. It is best to utilize fingerspelling sparingly because using it excessively can impede communication.

Conclusion

Gaining proficiency in ASL grammar and syntax necessitates an awareness of the language's peculiar characteristics and structure. This chapter explores the intricacies of role shifting, facial grammar, and advanced fingerspelling techniques, building on the groundwork established in previous sections.

Acquiring these sophisticated features of ASL grammar is about more than just learning the language; it's about developing a stronger bond with the Deaf community and the language itself. Richer and more complex communication is made possible by the opening up of new expressive and understanding aspects.

CHAPTER 2: UNDERSTANDING IDIOMS AND PHRASES IN ASL

Exploring American Sign Language (ASL) exposes a language environment full of colloquial terms and distinctive phrases that are as essential to the language as its individual signs. We'll delve into the intriguing realm of ASL idioms and phrases in this chapter. This investigation seeks to expand your awareness for the richness of ASL's language and culture in addition to improving your grasp of the language.

Like any language, ASL has its own collection of idiomatic expressions, which are statements that represent ideas or concepts that are understood by the Deaf community but do not transfer word for word into English. These expressions are crucial to fluent ASL communication because they frequently combine signs with non-manual cues like body language and facial expressions.

For instance, an ASL idiom like "TRAIN GONE SORRY" doesn't literally refer to a missed train. Instead, it's used to express the idea that you've missed out on what was being said or what's happening—akin to saying, "I've lost the thread of the conversation" in English. The sign for this idiom involves mimicking the movement of a train with your hands and then signing 'sorry,' accompanied by an appropriate facial expression.

Another interesting ASL idiom is "FINISH TOUCH," which is used to indicate that you're done dealing with something or someone. It's akin to saying "I'm done with it" in English. The signs involve miming the action of touching something and then showing completion.

Exploring idioms like "MIND OPEN" helps beginners understand the ASL approach to conceptual thinking. This phrase, which translates to "open-minded," involves signs that mimic opening something near the head, symbolizing an open mind. It's a great example of how ASL idioms can visually depict abstract concepts.

Idioms in ASL can also be culturally specific, providing insight into the Deaf community's experiences and perspectives. For example, the phrase "EYE PEOPLE," refers to the Deaf community itself, emphasizing the importance of visual communication and sight in Deaf culture. The sign for this idiom involves pointing to the eye and then gesturing to a group of people.

Understanding ASL phrases requires not only knowledge of the signs but also an understanding of the context in which they are used. For example, the phrase "CAN'T HEAR" in ASL doesn't always refer to the literal inability to hear. It's frequently used to convey miscommunication or a lack of comprehension. The sign involves shaking your head while signing 'hear,' indicating negation.

The nonliteral character of ASL idioms and phrases makes learning them difficult. In order to read the signs based on the context and the associated non-manual indicators, beginners must develop their visual and conceptual thinking skills. Compared to spoken languages, where idioms are typically comprehended by aural clues, this can be a very different way of thinking.

Immersion in ASL language and culture is essential for learning and applying ASL idioms and phrases successfully. Participating in Deaf community activities, interacting with native ASL speakers, and viewing ASL media can all offer invaluable opportunities to be exposed to these expressions in context. Furthermore, practicing these idioms with knowledgeable signers can provide you with understanding of their subtleties and application.

To sum up, ASL idioms and phrases are more than just linguistic peculiarities; they serve as entryways into the core of Deaf communication and culture. They give the language more nuance and cultural importance by layering on layers of meaning. Understanding and utilizing these idioms and phrases will help learners become more proficient in ASL and improve their capacity to communicate with the Deaf population.

In addition to being a crucial component of learning the language, this excursion into the complex world of ASL idioms and phrases is also an intriguing look into the diversity and ingenuity of Deaf culture. Accept these colloquial terms as essential parts of your language toolkit as you continue to study and use ASL, and take pleasure in the richer cultural connections they enable.

CHAPTER 3: FREQUENTLY ASKED QUESTIONS ABOUT LEARNING ASL

When learning American Sign Language (ASL), especially for the first time, many questions come up. The purpose of this chapter, "Frequently Asked Questions about Learning ASL," is to answer frequently asked questions with lucid, perceptive answers based on knowledge and experience from the actual world. We hope to increase your respect for and comprehension of ASL as we examine these questions, providing counsel that is consistent with this book's instructional objectives.

1. How long does it take to become fluent in ASL?

ASL proficiency varies based on a number of variables, such as practice frequency, exposure to native signers, and individual learning capacities. Fluency usually requires years of regular practice over several years, much like learning any other language.

2. Is ASL only used in the United States?

The US and some regions of Canada are the main countries where ASL is utilized. Different from ASL, several nations have their own sign languages, such as British Sign Language BSL in the UK.

3. Can learning ASL benefit my career?

Yes, learning ASL can greatly benefit your professional life, particularly if you work in public service, education, healthcare, or social work. It provides avenues for communication with the Deaf community and can be an advantageous ability in any line of work that involves interacting with customers.

4. What distinguishes conversational English from ASL?

ASL is a visual language with its own structure, rules of grammar, and construction unlike English. It conveys content by hand gestures, facial expressions, and body language. It also has a distinct phrase structure, frequently employing a "topic-comment" pattern.

5. What are the best ways to practice ASL?

Effective ways to practice include using internet resources like video tutorials, going to Deaf community events, and practicing with native ASL users. Complete immersion in the language and culture is necessary for better understanding and fluency.

6. Are there regional variations in ASL?

Indeed, ASL exhibits geographical differences and dialects, akin to spoken languages. The use of various signs for the same idea or phrase in various locales is one way to observe these variances.

7. To what extent do facial movements matter in ASL?

Expressions on the face are essential to ASL. They are necessary for efficient ASL communication because they can change the meaning of signals and offer emotional context.

8. Can I learn ASL by myself?

While independent study is an option, engaging with native signers and becoming immersed in the Deaf community are highly beneficial for learning ASL. Practicing in person is essential to becoming fluent.

9. What are some common challenges in learning ASL?

Adjusting to a visual-spatial language, comprehending the use of body language and facial emotions, and becoming used to the speed and fluidity of native signers are common obstacles.

10. How is ASL incorporated into the Deaf culture?

ASL is an integral component of Deaf culture, not just a tool for communication. It is essential to many Deaf people's identities and represents the community's ideals, experiences, and history.

11. Is ASL only for the Deaf?

No, a wide range of people, including hearing people, Deaf people's relatives, interpreters, and those wishing to communicate with the Deaf community, utilize ASL.

12. Can children learn ASL?

ASL is teachable to kids, and studies indicate that early exposure can improve language acquisition. Early acquisition of ASL is beneficial for both hearing and deaf youngsters.

13. How can I improve my ASL receptive skills?

ASL receptive skills can be improved with exposure and practice. You can improve your comprehension and interpretation of ASL by watching videos in the language, talking with native signers, and going to Deaf activities.

14. Are there any common misconceptions about ASL I should be aware of?

There is a widespread misperception that ASL is only signed English or that it is a universal language. Since ASL has its own grammar and syntax, not all Deaf people globally can understand it. It is a distinct language.

15. How does lip-reading complement ASL?

Even though ASL is a full language by itself, some Deaf and hard-of-hearing people also lip-read, particularly in situations when there is mixed communication. It's crucial to remember that everyone's lip-reading abilities differ significantly.

16. Can learning ASL help in understanding other sign languages?

Though each sign language has its own distinct structures and signs, learning ASL can give you a basic understanding of how sign languages function in general. Knowing ASL may not necessarily translate into understanding another sign language.

17. What are some effective strategies for learning ASL vocabulary?

Frequent practice, the use of visual aids, participating in ASL conversations, and the use of flashcards or applications specifically made for ASL learning can all help people acquire vocabulary in ASL more efficiently. Fluency in the language is essential.

18. How is storytelling done in ASL, and what makes it unique?

ASL storytelling is a colorful and expressive kind of art. Role-shifting, spatial utilization, classifiers, and expressive facial expressions are frequently used. ASL's visual-spatial characteristics provide for imaginative and captivating storytelling.

19. Are there any specific techniques to develop fluency in signing naturally and expressively?

Gaining proficiency in ASL requires consistent practice with native signers, comprehension of the subtle cultural differences in the language, and constant acquisition of new signs and expressions. It might also be beneficial to see and imitate the expressiveness and fluency of seasoned signers.

20. What resources are available for staying updated with new developments and changes in ASL?

Joining ASL clubs or online communities, watching ASL instructional videos, going to workshops, and taking part in Deaf community events are all ways to stay current. Updates and resources are also provided by numerous Deaf groups and colleges.

We hope to provide a thorough understanding of ASL, the learning process, and its role in the Deaf community by answering these commonly asked questions. This information improves your educational experience and strengthens your ties to ASL culture and language. Remember that every inquiry you ask and response you receive as you progress in learning ASL will bring you one step closer to gaining a deeper comprehension and respect of this wonderful language.

CHAPTER 4: REFLECTIONS ON YOUR ASL JOURNEY

It's crucial to take into account the road you've taken, the skills you've learned, and the cultural insights you've received when you look back on your journey to learn American Sign Language (ASL). Learning ASL is an intensive experience that opens doors to a lively cultural world and bridges linguistic boundaries, but it's much more than just picking up a new language.

It's likely that you were a little anxious and excited when you first started your adventure. Learning a new language, especially one as physically and spatially distinct as ASL, can be scary. It's possible that you began by learning the alphabet, rudimentary sentences, and signs. Even though they were difficult, these first steps set the groundwork for your ASL development.

As you progressed, you began to concentrate on learning the subtleties of facial expressions, comprehending the distinct grammar and sentence structure of ASL, and becoming used to the use of space in communication. The first time you realized you could follow a discussion in ASL or articulate your ideas clearly is a significant turning point in this journey. This development probably gave you a sense of accomplishment and increased your self-assurance in your ASL communication skills.

Immersion in the Deaf community and culture is a big part of learning ASL. An essential part of your journey is taking part in Deaf events, interacting with native ASL users, and learning about the experiences and history of the Deaf community. Along with improving language skills, this immersion helps people develop a greater appreciation and knowledge of the culture that ASL is a part of.

Every learning process has its share of difficulties, and it's possible that you had trouble understanding difficult ASL ideas, keeping up with native signers, or figuring out the subtle cultural differences within the Deaf community. Overcoming these challenges is one of the things that contributes importance to your knowledge. Overcoming obstacles is a step toward achieving not only language competency but also personal development and cultural awareness.

Because ASL and Deaf culture are closely related, learning ASL has probably given you a thorough understanding of Deaf culture. You now know that ASL is a language with its own idioms, sense of humor, and expressive ability, not just a handwritten version of English. As you've seen, ASL communication offers a rich, expressive, and extremely descriptive way of expression that goes beyond spoken words.

As you consider your past experiences, keep in mind that learning ASL is an ongoing process. There are constantly new things to discover, subtleties to grasp, and chances to strengthen your bonds with the Deaf community. Your future may involve developing your ASL abilities even further, standing up for the Deaf community, or even going into an area that deals with ASL and Deaf culture professionally.

Your efforts to learn ASL are evidence of your commitment and openness to a foreign language and way of life. It's a voyage that cuts over language barriers, deepens your comprehension of how people communicate, and ties you into a vibrant and varied group. Carry with you the knowledge, abilities, and cultural understanding you have received as you proceed down this path, and anticipate the many more pleasant encounters that await you on your never-ending journey with ASL.

CHAPTER 5: BONUS: TIPS FOR FAST AND EFFECTIVE LEARNING

The rich, complicated lexicon of American Sign lexicon (ASL) requires both physical dexterity and mental comprehension. Learning ASL involves more than just learning signs; it also involves accepting a new way of communicating that combines body language, facial expressions, and hand gestures.

1. Spaced Repetition: A Strategic Approach to Long-term Retention

The "forgetting curve," which implies that human memory retention is better each time we review knowledge after a period of forgetting, is the theoretical foundation for spaced repetition. Increasing the time between practice sessions is like teaching your brain to remember sign language information for extended periods of time.

Advanced Use: You might want to practice signals associated with everyday tasks in the morning and review them in the evening. Stretch this time out across a few days and weeks at a time. This method is especially helpful for maintaining the finer points of ASL, like the minute differences in hand forms or motions that might alter a sign's meaning.

2. Elaborative Interrogation: Enhancing Understanding Through Inquiry

The goal of this approach is to comprehend the logic and structure of the language in order to develop a deeper relationship with it. To indicate "more" in ASL, for instance, tap your fingertips together. Reminding yourself that this is a symptom of wanting more of something will help you remember it.

Exercise for Practice: Whenever you come across a new sign, spend a few minutes learning about its history and many use. This could be observing videos of ASL users who are native speakers or asking teachers about the subtleties of the sign.

3. Active Learning: Immersion and Interaction

Passive observation is not the only way to learn actively. It's important to fully ingrain the language. This could be going to social gatherings for the Deaf community, joining sign language groups, or even doing volunteer work in Deaf areas.

Practical Use: Consider recounting your everyday activities in ASL. This exercise helps with vocabulary practice as well as knowing how ASL sentences are structured, which is different from English sentences in many ways. For example, a topic-comment sentence structure is frequently used in ASL, which is an important concept to understand for efficient communication.

4. Practice Testing: Self-Assessment in ASL

ASL practice exams involve more than just repeating signs. It's important to comprehend the subtle differences between each sign, the syntax that connects them, and the phrases that provide meaning. There are several ways to regularly evaluate yourself:

- **Online Quizzes**: There are several websites with quizzes designed especially for people learning ASL. These can include everything from reading signs to interpreting sentences between ASL and English.
- **Study Partners**: Practice with a partner to get quick feedback. It also aids in comprehending the potential appearance of signs from the viewpoint of the recipient, an often neglected facet of learning sign language.
- **Video Recording**: Making a video of your own signature and playing it back works wonders. It enables you to recognize and correct mistakes in your hand patterns, facial gestures, and overall fluency.

In-Depth Example: Try writing down a brief story in ASL, either a retelling of a beloved tale or a daily journal entry. Watch and record, noting areas that need work, such as the appropriateness of facial expressions, the smoothness of sign transitions, and the clarity of the signs. Compare these recordings over time to track your development.

5. Interleaving: Mixing It Up

Creating a varied learning environment in each session is the goal of interleaving in ASL instruction. Combine various categories of indicators rather than concentrating on just one (such as just emotions or colors). It has been demonstrated that this method enhances memory as well as information application skills in various situations.

Expanded Practical Tip: Practice signing a story with multiple aspects in a single session. For example, a story about visiting a park could have symbols for the colors green grass, blue sky, and happiness, excitement, and walking and playing. This form of exercise improves general ASL fluency by teaching your brain to adapt and learn to switch between several sign languages and concepts.

6. Visualization and Mnemonics: Creating Mental Links

Because ASL is primarily visual, visualization and mnemonics are very helpful in education. Memorization can be greatly aided by associating a tale or mental image with the motion or form of a sign.

- **For the sign "tree"**: Consider a tree that is blown by the wind. The fingers stand in for waving branches, and the arm depicts the trunk. Because it resembles the real tree movement, this graphic aids in remembering the symbol.
- **For the sign "book"**: Imagine that a book is opened. The hands that are opening in front of you resemble a book cover being opened. This aids with both recalling the sign and comprehending its meaning, as many ASL signals are based on tangible or visual metaphors.

Advanced Mnemonics Example: To help you recall the advanced mnemonics for "butterfly," you may imagine or write a short story about a butterfly flapping its wings, which is similar to the hand motion in the sign. This aids in both recalling the symbol and connecting it to the elegant, fluttering movement of a butterfly.

7. Self-Explanation: Teaching Yourself

One useful technique for learning ASL is self-explanation. It entails a more in-depth interaction with the language, going beyond simple mimicry to a thorough comprehension of all the intricacies and variations of each sign.

Extensive Practice: After mastering the sign for "friend," for instance, dissect each component of the sign. Observe how the intertwined index fingers signify a connection or bond—a crucial component of friendship. "In what contexts can I use this sign?" ask yourself. Is it suitable in both formal and informal contexts?" These types of questions improve memory retention and help you gain a deeper knowledge of ASL's expressive potential.

8. Optimized Study Environment

One of the most important factors in learning ASL is the learning environment. Because ASL is a visual language, your learning area needs to be set up so that you can practice and observe precise hand and facial gestures.

Establishing the Perfect Environment: Make sure there is enough light in your study space so you can see hand movements and forms properly. Reduce the amount of auditory distractions—which, even when learning a visual language, may be quite disruptive. A mirror can help you notice and adjust your facial expressions and sign formations, which are essential for communicating meaning in ASL.

9. Time Management: The Pomodoro Technique

Time management skills are critical, especially when learning a language as tactile and visually demanding as ASL. The Pomodoro Technique is particularly useful for avoiding weariness and helping you stay focused.

How to Use the Technique: Set a timer for 25 minutes of focused practice using ASL. After that, take a 5-minute break. To avoid strain, rest your hands and eyes during these periods. In addition to improving focus, interval training guarantees that you practice consistently without becoming exhausted.

10. Practical Application: Using ASL in Real Life

The ability to use a language in everyday situations is the final test of any language acquisition process. The same is true with ASL. Interacting with the Deaf population or applying ASL in real-world contexts greatly improves your educational experience.

Real-Life Application: Participate in ASL meet-up groups or attend Deaf social gatherings. Engage in sign language practice with Deaf people to enhance your skills and gain understanding of the subtle cultural differences in the language. To simulate real-life conversations, use video calls to practice ASL with other students or proficient signers.

Gaining proficiency in ASL involves interacting with a lively community and culture. You improve both your signing and your knowledge of Deaf culture by using these comprehensive and varied learning options. Recall that mastering ASL involves more than just picking up the language—it involves adopting a rewarding cultural experience.

CHAPTER 6: CONCLUSIONS

As this guide to learning American Sign Language (ASL) draws to a close, it's important to pause and consider the trip thus far. ASL is more than just a language; with its diverse range of gestures, facial expressions, and body language, it offers access to a lively community and an alternative perspective on the outside world.

ASL's complexity and beauty are highlighted by its unusual structure, which sets it apart from spoken languages. Unlike just translating English words into signs, ASL is a unique language with its own structure, rules of grammar, and cultural contexts. This knowledge is essential because it enables us to recognize the language's significance for the identity and culture of the Deaf community.

Accepting ASL also entails accepting the culture and people of the Deaf community. This path is about more than just learning a new language; it's about appreciating and comprehending a rich cultural history. As students, we join a larger story that promotes diversity and inclusivity.

The way we learn ASL has changed dramatically since the advent of technology. Learning has become more accessible thanks to digital tools, internet resources, and apps, which offer chances for practice, repetition, and interaction. It's imperative to strike a balance between these virtual encounters and practice and real-world interactions. In lieu of true involvement with the language and the Deaf community, technology ought to be a supplement.

Difficulties are a given when learning ASL. It's a language requiring not just mental comprehension but also dexterity and physical aptitude. Never lose sight of the fact that studying a language is something that requires patience and plenty of time. You get more fluent with every sign you learn and every linguistic detail you comprehend. The journey is just as satisfying as the destination, and each obstacle you overcome is evidence of your commitment and diligence.

In the future, mastering ASL will be an ongoing effort. The language's evolution reflects the dynamic nature of both the Deaf community and society at large. Maintaining and improving your talents requires participation in continuing education, staying involved in the community, and staying up to date with new advancements.

In summary, the following are important takeaways:

- **Learn the fundamentals**: Fluency is built on a foundation of basic signs and grammar.
- **Practice frequently and in different contexts**. This will assist you in remembering what you've studied and improving your proficiency with ASL's nuances.
- **Get fully absorbed in the culture**: Engaging with the Deaf community improves your comprehension and ability.
- **Make sensible use of technology**: Let digital tools support, not take over, your educational journey.

Being an ASL master is a rewarding journey, not a race, so be patient and persistent.

We should stress the fundamental nature of this book as you go on your path to learn American Sign Language (ASL) as we consider its content and organization. Carefully crafted, this book seeks to offer the most thorough and reliable starting point for those just starting out on their ASL learning journey.

Our strategy has been to fully cover the fundamentals, from syntax and basic indicators to cultural quirks and real-world applications. Because each chapter is designed to build upon the one before it, the learning curve is rational and progressive. All of the activities, examples, and helpful hints are designed to help you learn the language and gain a deeper comprehension of its cultural background.

But it's important to recognize that no single book can capture the richness and diversity of American Sign Language (ASL) because of its immensity and constant evolution. Like any language, ASL is a dynamic system that develops over time. While this guide covers a wide array of topics and provides a solid foundation, it is just the beginning of a lifelong journey of learning and exploration.

This book is structured to be as complete and comprehensive as possible within the confines of a single volume. Our intention has been to encourage you to keep learning after reading these pages by providing you with the essential information and tools needed to communicate successfully in ASL. As you explore the world of ASL, keep in mind that this book is just a beginning point—a manual for the principles—upon which you can expand your knowledge and abilities.

In the beginning of your ASL adventure, consider this book to be your devoted companion. It establishes the foundation, provides entry to novel experiences, and sets you on the route to fluency and a more profound comprehension of other cultures. Acquiring proficiency in ASL is a rewarding and demanding endeavor, and this guide aims to provide you with the most robust and thorough foundation possible. To keep improving your ASL skills and appreciation, be inquisitive, look for new opportunities to learn, and get involved in the Deaf community.

In the end, it's critical to keep in mind that learning ASL, like learning any language, is a process that calls for persistence, patience, and time. The difficulties shouldn't deter you; they are a necessary component of learning. You may unlock a new realm of understanding and communication by becoming proficient in ASL with dedication and persistence. Although the path may be lengthy, there are incalculable benefits to interacting with the Deaf population and adopting a different cultural viewpoint. As you proceed down this route, acknowledge your accomplishments at every turn and realize that you are making the world a more welcoming and varied place with every sign you learn.

Made in the USA
Las Vegas, NV
17 January 2024

84321565R10059